INTRODUCTION TO MIDWIFERY

Dr. Sathiyalatha Sarathi

RIGI PUBLICATION

INTRODUCTION TO MIDWIFERY

By

Dr. Sathiyalatha Sarathi

Originally published in India

Edition: 1

ISBN: 978-93-91041-84-7

Published by RIGI PUBLICATION

777, Street no.9, Krishna Nagar Khanna-141401 (Punjab), India

Website: www.rigipublication.com

Email: info@rigipublication.com

Phone: +91-9357710014, +91-9465468291

PREFACE

Nurses and Midwives contribute a major role in health care delivery system and easily accessible to people seeking health care, are better aware of their problems and are in position to understand the complex nature of the heath care of health care provision, especially of reproductive health. They have shown great flexibility, innovation and commitment in shaping and developing new roles and services which are aimed to reducing Maternal mortality and improving maternal care.

This textbook includes Historical perspectives of Midwifery in India, Milestones of Midwifery, current perspectives of Maternal and child health services including recent Maternal and Child Health (MCH) Schemes, Maternal Mortality and its preventive strategies, Ethics and standards of midwifery practice including code of ethics by Indian Nursing council. Also, incorporated with scope of practice for Midwives, Trends in Midwifery including recent trends in obstetrics and Gynecology, Evidence based Nursing& Midwifery practice. In addition, Genetics and Genetic counselling are incorporated.

I have endeavored to provide sustained knowledge to students on Midwifery and different aspects of Midwifery and Obstetrical Nursing and hope that they will find this book to be a good resource of midwifery practice. I thank my beloved teacher Dr. A.V Raman, imparted me the knowledge regarding Maternal Nursing which helps me to compile this book.

Dr. Sathiyalatha Sarathi

CONTENTS

1. HISTORICAL PERSPECTIVES OF MIDWIFERY IN INDIA

Midwifery is an old profession, and typically a feminine occupation, traditionally passed down in the family and involved intimate social relationships between midwife and women in birth process. Early attempts of teaching and learning midwifery began at the end of medieval period and increased during 18th and 19th centuries. The history of midwifery demonstrates the authority during childbirth in ancient period and later changed based on availability of obstetric services.

History of midwifery in India:

The word midwife means **"with women"**. Midwives are described by as special people with special attributes, wise women. Her skill is based on a mixture of art and science. Art, it requires her to able to understand the women's needs, to encourage her and build her confidence. Science, it requires higher degree of knowledge. The midwife applies these art and science in her practice that is the reason that midwife it said to be the **"wise women"**. The major role of the midwife is the satisfactory provision of maternal and childcare.

In India, maternal and childcare perspectives are described in three periods.

* **Ancient period to before the British India**

* **During the time of British India**

* **After the British India (or) Independent India**

Ancient India to before the British India

In ancient India, care of women and practice of midwifery were totally in the hands of indigenous village dais. Even today majority of deliveries in rural india are being conducted by dais.

The occupation of dais is was hereditary. It passed from mother and daughters or to daughters-in-law. They belonged to lower caste.

Childbirth was considered a time of impurity. As such, the worst room in the household was selected delivery and those belonging to lower castes could only attend a woman during childbirth.

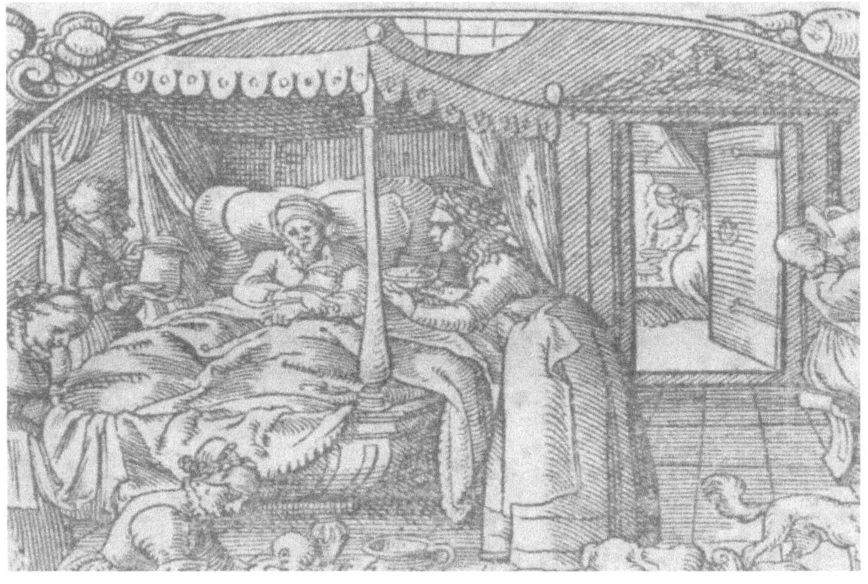

Figure 1: Historical Horror of Childbirth

Dais gained their skill through observation and practice. This knowledge of the process of childbirth was based on what they saw and experience. No formal training was given.

Traditional practices of untrained TBAs include such procedure such as

---

***Adjusting the position of the foetus.**
***Massaging the abdomen of the pregnant women.**

***Advising on diet**

***Administering medicine**

During the initial stage of labour, the TBA wash her hands. The pregnant woman iss fed which is thought the booster her strength during labour and help to speed up the delivery. The mother is encouraged to walk around the room. Vaginal palpation is used to determine how soon and how fast the baby is coming.

The position the mother assumes during the actual delivery depends upon previous experiences or local traditions. Possible positions include kneeling, reclining, sitting over a basin, stunting or suspension by the armpits

The infant is received in a clean cloth. Eyes, ears, nose and mouth are washed with warm water. To stimulate respiration the baby is fanned with a cloth and slapped on the buttocks and chest.

Various instruments are used to the umbilical cord: such as sharp-edged instruments, knife etc. A strong thread in used to tie the umbilical cord.

The criteria used to decide where to cut the umbilical cord vary with traditions of each community. Some examples are

---

***For boy babies, 3 finger length is measured. It is believed that anything over this length will make the baby grow up to a scoundrel. (Rogue)**

***For girl babies, a hand's breath is used and shorter, that the girl will be too narrow in the hips.**

In some places, the distance from the tip of the outstretched thump to that of the index finger about 12-15cm is measured off for both boys and girls. With less than that a girl might have a small uterus.

If the placenta is not expelled immediately a receptacle with heated brandy may place close to vagina to loosen the afterbirths (placenta and umbilical cord, placental membrane). The mother may be made to shallow a raw egg or almond oil. And less she is haemorrhaging, the mother is sometimes rubbed with belladonna leaves and bound tightly in sheets from waist to knee for 3days. This procedure is believed to help the pelvic bones resume their normal position.

After the birth, the mother is encouraged to have had special bath in which the water would be mixed with herbs to help her feel fresh and energetic.

As long as it was normal delivery and everything went smoothly, they did not have a problem. Their presence was more than the support gave. The childbirth rituals and practices are also practiced by cleaning, fireworks flowers, and gifts etc.

But when they came across the case of complications, the dais could not handle the situation and serious morbidity and mortality were the result. Fatalistic and supernatural explanations had to be sought to explain these "beyond human control" phenomena.

The period of British India:

At the end of the 19th century and at the beginning of the 20th century the health of the public become a major concern, when it was found that facilities to meet the health needs of the Indian population.

The initiative to meet these needs began in 1871. Miss. Hewlett, Ms. Pricilla Winter, Deaconess Faltz and Deaconess Bielbly are the well-known "sisters" who came to India to train nurse at the request of the government of madras. As early as in 1877 Miss Hewett, an English woman who started English missionary society which was the first training school for dais in Amritsar.

In 1875, Ms. Elizabeth Bielby has reported to queen victories about her observation regarding the lack of health services to mother and children especially during pregnancy and child birth. The queen has entrusted Lady Dufferin with the task of providing medical services to the women in India..

In 1885 Mrs. Dufferin established "National association" for providing medical aid to the Indian women by collecting the resources both from England and India. During this movement, Dias were properly identified as the best links for better results. Hence the Dias training has become a vital source in midwifery. Mrs. Hewlett started regular class in 1885 for Dias in Amritsar and paid some amount of money for regular attendance in classes and gave certificate after a short training programme. She personally supervised the care given by Dias and if satisfied, paid them one rupee per case which she has received from Amritsar municipality. Thus safe home delivery was able to be provided. Similar services were provided in other provinces also with the help of Dufferin fund.

In 1900 Dias training programme was taken up by "Provincial Government" with the provision of Victoria Memorial scholarship fund which was established by Lady Curzan.

In 1918 Ms. Griffin and Miss. Graham were appointed at Delhi and they contributed much for the development of child welfare. In 1919, Lady Chelmsford gave more importance for child welfare services. In 1920, maternal and child welfare exhibition was organized through the efforts of the the "Dufferin Association".

The Indian Red Cross society took interest in the work which was started by the "Chelmsford league" for maternal and child welfare.

The baby week movement was started by Lady Reading. Later this initiative took a momentum and "Baby weeks" were organized throughout India.

Ms. Griffin and Ms. Graham jointly started a school for health visitors in Delhi near Kashmiri gate. Later, a building at Bara Hindu Rao was given to them by the kindness of Lady Reading. Her school become the present "Lady Reading health school".

Since dais were unable to deal with difficult deliveries and pregnancies, the maternal and neonatal mortality were very high in British India.,

When medical missionary women such as Miss Ethel Bleakly and Miss Edith Simpson were noticed that the, the infant mortality rate was 400 per thousand. In one village they heard that ten babies born had all died one after the other due to tetanus. They had been attended to by the "same dais".

A missionary doctor wrote in 1927, states that ignorance and malpractice in abnormal midwifery cases in the major cause of high infant mortality rate in India.

1918, Lady Reading health school even established at Delhi to train health visitors for providing public health services, maternal and child health services and to supervise axillary nurse midwifes. This was another steppingstone in the maternal child health services.

1921: Lady Chelmsford league was formed in India developing maternity and child welfare services.

1926: The Madras presidency always wanted nurse midwives and train a superior class of midwife. The state succeeded in doing so by in challenging the Madras registration of nurses and midwives act, 1926 to promote a registered midwives for service during childbirth.

1931: The Indian Red Cross society established MCH bureau in association with the lady Chelmsford leagues and Victoria memorial scholarship fund are coordinate the MCH work throughout the country. Madras was the first state to setup a separate section of maternal and child welfare in the public health. Again, madras was the first state to attempt to replace dais by the better qualified personal, such as midwives and Nurse-midwives.

1936: Dufferin fund sanctioned which are used to increase the number of Dufferin hospitals, to build hostels, supply teaching materials and employ qualified sister in nursing schools. The Dufferin fund thus helped in raising the standards of nursing and midwifery in the country.

1938: Indian Research Fund association was established which had a committee that undertook the investigation about the incidence and causes of maternal and infant morbidity and mortality.

Sir. A.L Mudaliar was the key person of the committee. Investigation thus carried out in certain sites of the country revealed that

a. **Institutional midwifery services were limited**
b. **Maternal and child welfare services were poorly equipped and staffed**
c. **Deliveries were mostly handled by untrained dais.**

This situation continued for some more time.

In 1946 the bore committee (Health survey and development committee), in this famous report urged a very high priority for MCH services in the development of health services in India. The Bhore committee reported a very high maternal mortality rate in India. 20 per 1000 live births in 1938. The committee recommended that the health services for mother and children should also included. The grant of maternity leave with benefit for a period of 6 weeks before and 6weeks after confinement for all working women also formed.

MCH services in Independent India:

In 1947: Independence causes tremendous changes in nursing education in the country. The first step that the Indian nursing council, took after its inspection in 1947, was to combine the nursing and midwifery courses into a single course. The course was designed to be of 3 ½ years duration, with entry qualification of being class X.

The second change brought about in newly independent India was to replace the diploma in midwifery course, by an auxiliary nursing and midwifery (ANM) course of 2 year with the basic qualification being class VIII. These auxiliary nurse midwives wear specially trained in midwifery and childcare services in order to be posted at primary health centres, mainly to look after mother and children and conduct deliveries.

1952: INC emphasized and developed a curriculum for general nursing and integration of public health nurse in general nurse midwife.

1953: The center council of health as its first meeting in January 1953 had recommended the establishment of primary health centers. After this period PHC are started to develop.

1950: Dr. Ida Scudder, trained women doctors for maternal and childcare in CMCH Vellore.

1955: Shetty committee appointed by the government of India, recommended training, and posting ANM, in health centres for maternal and childcare services.

1959: Bischoff, a technical consultant who recommended the two types of nursing personnel- the auxiliary nurse midwife and the general nurse midwife.

In 1975: The popular Kartar Singh committee recommended multipurpose health workers scheme, thereby the two year ANM course was shortened by 6 months and a broad curriculum was designed providing a wide range of experiences in community health. The entry requirement was class X.

The multipurpose health workers work is focused:

- **Center to primary**
- **Uni-purpose to multipurpose**
- **Specialization to generalization**
- **Global to local**
- **Curative to preventive**

1983: The national health plan (1983) proposed re-organization of primary health centres on the basis of PHC for every 30,000 rural population in the plains, and one PHC for every 20,000-population in hilly, tribal and backward areas for more effective coverage. The sub centres established on the basis of 5000 population in general and one for every 3000 population in hilly, tribal and backward areas. Each PHC has 16 sub centres. The sub centre should have one male and female health workers. In PHC there will be 4 male and female MPHW.

1992: The Child survival and safe motherhood (CSSM) programme was launched on August 1992. This programme was specially designed for maternal and child health services.

1997: Improving maternal and child health has been one of the top priorities of the Government of India. The reproductive and child health (RCH) Programme – Phase 1 was launched on 15th October,1997. This RCH programme – Phase 1 has essential activities.

- Identification of the pregnant mothers under coverage of PHC
- 100% registration of pregnant mothers.
- 100% coverage of TT vaccine to pregnant mothers

- Minimum three visits during pregnancy
- Delivery by the health professionals. In home setup delivery must be conducted by trained
- health workers female.
- 100% registration of the newborn.
- 100% birth weight record should be maintained.
- 10% high risk newborn must be referred.
- Immunization
- Emphasis on family planning.

While countries in the west are moving in the direction of specialized courses coutries for professional midwifery practice, independent midwifery practitioners and team midwifery practice. Our country stays behind to deliver skilled services to women in labour. Midwifery has to stop being a branch of nursing or an appendage of obstetrics and develop as an independent practice in the health care delivery system in order to better the midwifery procedures to the most comfortable, safe and satisfying childbirth.

Milestones in Midwifery:

Hippocrates (460BC), the further of scientific medicine, organized, trained and supervised midwives. However, his method was crude, Hippocrates did not contribute much of midwifery. He believed that the fetus had to fight its way out of the womb and that the bones of pelvic girdle separated during the process of childbirth. The effort of Hippocrates, any way not appreciated by the midwives.

Aristotle(384-322BC), the father of embryology, described the uterus and the pelvic organs. He also discussed the essential qualities of midwife. Celsus (30AD) published 'De medicina', he was first to propose an internal podalic version of a dead fetus. Soranus (second century AD) was the first to specialize in obstetrics and gynaecology. His book remained the best for 1500 years. He used a vaginal speculum and advised on cord care and wet nursing.

Leonardo da Vinci(1452-1519) made anatomical drawings which showed a pregnant uterus with breech presenting foetus inside. In 1953, the first book of midwifery was printed in Germany, based on 'Soranus' teaching. In 1940, it was translated into English as 'Ye Byrth of Mankind'. Vasalius (1543), opened a full-term pregnant uterus and extracted the foetus- an experimental caesarean section. He demonstrated the uterus as a single chamber organ.

Ambroise Pare (1510-1590) laid the foundations of modern obstetrics. He reintroduced internal podalic version, which he had learnt from Hery and Lembart, Master Barbeo surgeons in Paris. His skill in delivering the child alive enhanced his prestige among midwives. He was the first to deliver a woman in bed, instead of in a birth stool. He also sutured perineal tears. He founded a school for midwives in Paris.

Louise Bourgeois, recommended induction of labour for pelvic contraction. Julius Caessar Aranzi wrote the first text book for Italian midwives, which ran 17 editions. He advised caesarean section for a contracted pelvis.

William Harvey,(1578-1657), the father of British midwifery, wrote the first English text book of Midwifery. He described the placenta and the foetal circulation. He was the first person to deliver the placenta by kneading the uterus. He described raw placental bed surface and this initiated the study uterine sepsis.

Mauriceau was the greatest Obstetrician of 17th century. He described the attitude of foetus in the uterus. Chamberlin(1697-1763) designed obstetric forceps. William Smellie (1697-1763) was called father of British midwifery. He showed labour to be a mechanical process. He showed labour to be a mechanical process. He described Pelvimetry and cephalometry, diagonal conjugate, rachitic and contracted pelvis and forceps delivery of the aftercoming head of a breech. He devised a lock for obstetric forceps, which permitted to be inserted separately.

Justin Siegemund(1636-1705) was a renowned midwife who explained in detail about breech delivery. The image is from a **book Court Midwife,** her book was published in 1690, was the first German medical text written by a woman.

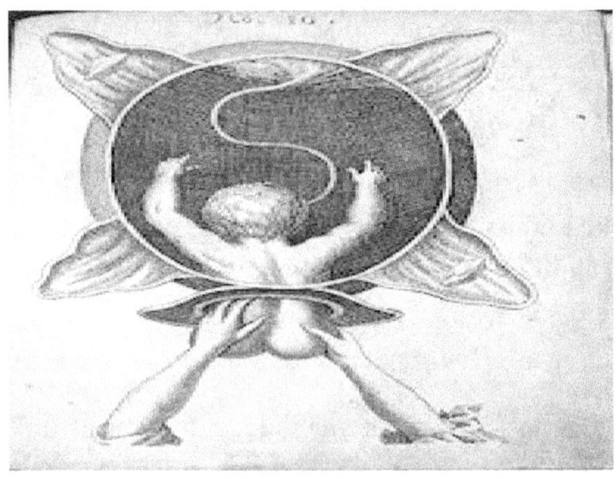

Figure 2: Image of Breech Delivery from the Book Court Midwife

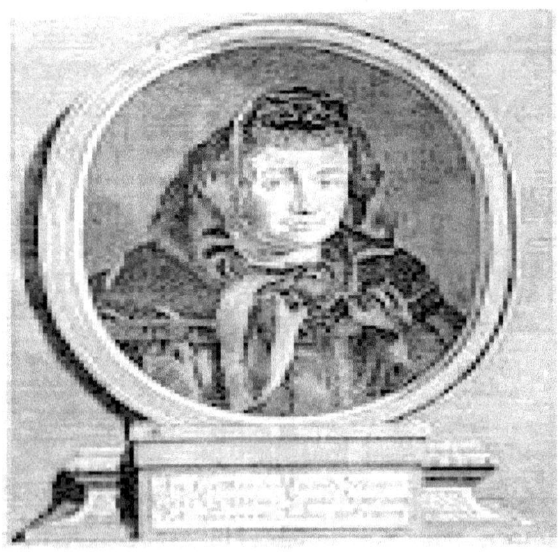

Figure 3: Justin Siegemund renowned German Midwife (1636-1705)

Charles white (1773) stated first that puerperal fever was infections. He used lime as disinfectant. Sigault (1777) described the operation of symphysiotomy. Fielding Ould (1710-1789) described the mechanism of labour, and performed the first episiotomy. Gordon (1795) showed that puerperal sepsis was a wound contamination of the placental site. Oliver Wendall Holmes (1843) wrote a treatise on puerperal fever.

Francois mayor (1818) first recognized foetal heart sounds in the pregnant uterus, but their importance was recognized by his pupil kergaredee while listening for splashing sounds made by the fetus in the amniotic fluid.

James young Simpson (1847) used chloroform first in obstetrics for anaesthesia. Florence Nightingale was a pioneer in the efficient training of midwives. In 1862 she organized a small training school in connection with king's college Hospital.

James young Simpson (1847) used chloroform first in obstetrics for anaesthesia. Florence Nightingale was a pioneer in the efficient training of midwives. In 1862 she organized a small training school in connection with king's college Hospital.

Ignaz Semmelweis (1818-1865) known as **Father of Infection control**. Dr. Ignaz Semmelweis demonstrated the cause of puerperal sepsis, and suggested prevention for the same. His contribution in midwifery services emphasized the importance of hygienic practices during delivery and postnatal period. Hand hygiene is noted to be the single most important factor for infection control. He observed that women delivered by physicians and medical students had a much higher rate (13–18%) of post-delivery mortality (called puerperal fever or childbed fever) than women delivered by midwife trainees or midwives (2%) in Allgemeine Krankenhaus teaching hospital in Vienna (1844). So, he is more appreciated among midwives and called as 'Saviour of Mothers.

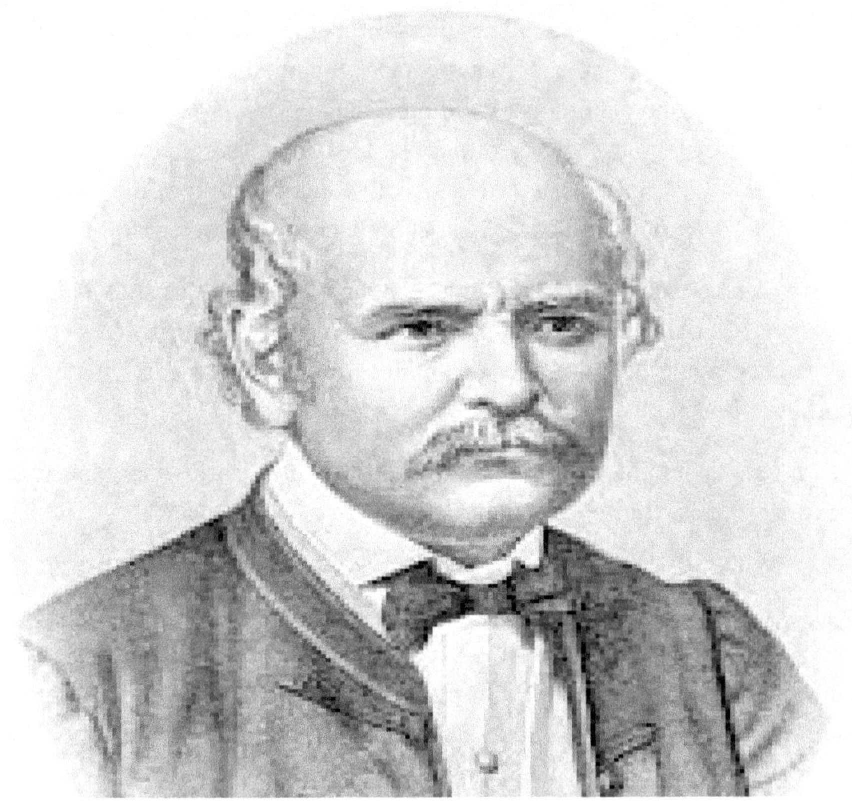

Figure 4: Ignaz Semmelweis (1818 -1865) "Saviour of Mothers"

Professor Herbert Spencer (1901) suggested external cephalic version for a breech in the antenatal period, using pinard's method, at about 30th week of pregnancy.

I have endeavoured to outline a few of the most notable advances in the practice of the obstetric art during the past 450 years, and in particular to give some insight into a few of the remarkable men responsible for planting firmly these important milestones. I have made no mention of antenatal pathology and physiology, for these are of such recent development that nearly all our knowledge of them has accrued within the limits of the present century. That is undoubtedly the field with which all modern workers are chiefly concerned, and it is in that field that the next important milestone will be founded

REFERENCE:

1. Kasturi Sundar Rao, An introduction to community Health Nursing.
2. Susan Klein, A manual for trained birth attendants and community midwives.
3. Jaqueline Vincent priya, Birth without doctors.
4. Park J.E, Essentials of community Health Nursing.
5. Park, Preventive, and social medicine.
6. Grace Paul N.Rao, History of Nursing.
7. Dr. Shashank V. Paurlkar, Textbook for Midwives.
8. Reena Bose & Prakassama, Midwifery in India: Past, Present and Future.
9. Spencer. *Br Med J* 1901; **1:1192**–6.
10. Milestones in Midwifery. http://pmj.bmj.com

2. CURRENT PRESPECTIVES OF MATERNAL AND CHILD HEALTH SERVICES RECENT MCH SCHEME

Reproductive and child health (RCH) – Phase II:

The second phase of RCH program i.e. RCH-II was launched on 1st April,2005. The main objective of the program was to bring about a change in mainly three indicators. These are reducing total fertility rate, infant mortality rate and maternal mortality rate to achieve the outcomes envisioned in the millennium Developmental goals.

The aim RCH Program is to reduce the maternal morbidity and mortality and promote adolescent health.

Components of RCH

- **Essential Obstetrical care**
- **Emergency Obstetrical care**
- **Strengthening Infrastructure**
- **Capacity Building**
- **Improving referral system**
- **Innovative Schemes**

Essential Obstetrical Care:
- Promotion of Institutional deliveries.
- 50% of the Primary centres and Community health centres made operational as 24hours delivery centres.
- Skilled attendance at birth.
- Policy decisions to permit health workers to use drugs in emergency situations to reduce maternal mortality.

Operationalization of FRUs (First Referral Units) to provide:

- 24 hours delivery services.
- Emergency Obstetric Care.
- Safe abortion services.
- Emergency care of the sick child.
- Treatment of RTI and STI.
- Blood storage facility
- Essential laboratory services.
- Referral transport system.

RECENT MCH SCHEMES:

Maternal Health is a vital parameter for assessing the quality of health services in a country. Maternal Mortality Ratio is used for recording maternal health status of a community. It is defined as the number of maternal deaths per 100,000 live births from any cause related to or aggravated by pregnancy or its management and not due to accidental or incidental causes. In the end of the last decade, Maternal Mortality Ratio (MMR) in India was pegged at 556 per lakh live births. In 2000 it stood at 374 per lakh live births. Subsequently, in the year 2011-2013 it declined to 167 and currently in 2015 it stands at 130 per lakh live births. The decline has been most profound in Empowered Action Group (EAG) states namely Uttar Pradesh, Uttarakhand, Madhya Pradesh, Chhattisgarh, Bihar, Jharkhand, Rajasthan, Odisha. This remarkable pace of decline can be attributed to the government of India schemes aimed at improving maternal health. In this writeup the currently implemented various government of India schemes for improving maternal health have been discussed.

Recent approaches In Maternal and childcare in India:

---

1. **RMNCH+Approach**
2. **Janani Surekha Yojana.**
3. **MCH Wings.**
4. **Capacity Building.**
5. **Training ASHS & ANMs.**
6. **MCTs Tracking**
7. **National Iron Plus Initiative.**
8. **Dakshata Guidelines**

RMNCH+A approach

- RMNCH+A approach has been launched in 2013 and it essentially looks to address the major causes of mortality among women and children as well as delay in accessing and utilizing healthcare and services.
- The RMNCH+A approach has been developed to provide an understanding of continuum care to ensure equal focus on various life strategies.
- Maternal health – interventions
- Use MCTS
- High risk pregnancies
- Review maternal and Infant deaths
- Identify low institutional delivery areas and incentivize ANMs for domiciliary

Janani Suraksha Yojana(JSV)

- The scheme focuses on identifying poor pregnant women in low performing states(LPS)- Utter Pradesh, Uttaranchal, Bihar, Jharkhand, Madhya Pradesh, Chhattishgarh, Assam, Rajasthan, Orissa and Jammu and Kashmir.

- Tracking each Pregnancy: Each beneficiary registered under the Yojana should have a JSV card and along with MCH Card. ASHA/AWW/ under the supervision of ANM and MO, should mandatorily prepare the micro-birth plan. This will effectively help in monitoring Ante-natal Check-ups and the post delivery care.

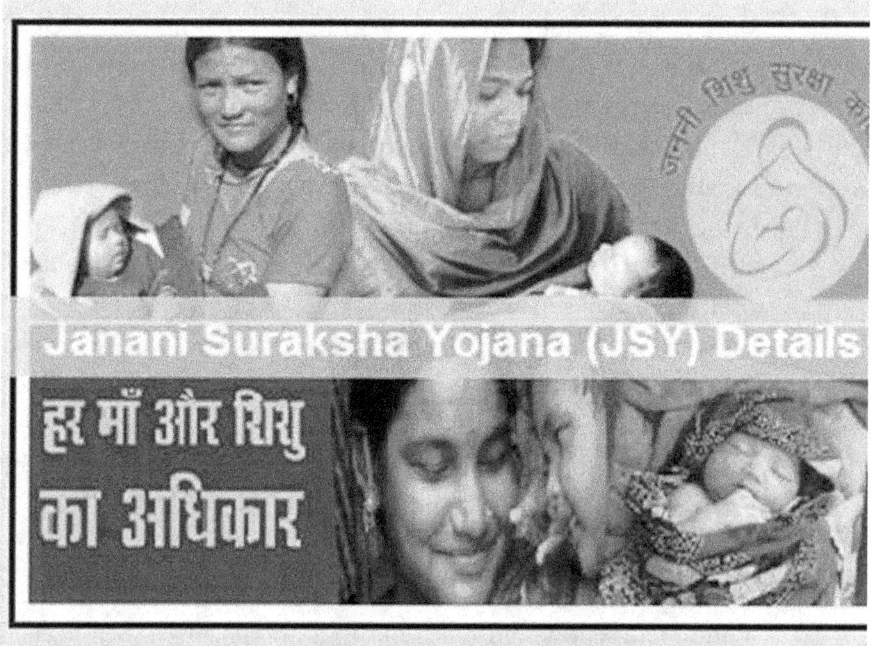

Figure 5: Janani Suraksha Yojana

Pradhan Mantri Surakshit Matritva Abhiyan (PMSMA)

- The Pradhan Mantri Surakshit Matritva Abhiyan(PMSMA) has been launched by the Ministry of Health & Family Welfare (MoHFW) in June, 2016.
- Rational for the program:
- Data indicates that Maternal Mortality Ratio (MMR) in India was very high in the year 1990 with 556 women dying during

- childbirth per hundred thousand live births as compared to the global MMR of 385/lakh live births.
- As per RGI- SRS (2011-13), MMR of India has now declined to 167/lakh live births against a global MMR of 216/lakh live births (2015).
- India has registered an overall decline in MMR of 70% between 1990 and 2015 in comparison to a global decline of 44%.
- Antenatal checkup services would be provided by OBGY specialists / Radiologist/physicians with support from private sector doctors to supplement the efforts of the government sector.
- A minimum package of antenatal care services (including investigations and drugs) would be provided to the beneficiaries on the 9th day of every month at identified public health facilities (PHCs/ CHCs, DHs/ urban health facilities etc) in both urban and rural areas.
- Using the principles of a single window system, it is envisaged that a minimum package of investigations (including one ultrasound during the 2nd trimester of pregnancy) and medicines such as IFA supplements, calcium supplements etc would be provided to all pregnant women attending the PMSMA clinics.

PMSMA- Mother Child Protection (MCP) Cards

- While the target would reach out to all pregnant women special efforts would be made to reach out to women who have not registered for ANC (left out/missed ANC) and also those who have registered but not availed ANC services (dropout) as well as High Risk pregnant women.
- OBGY specialists/ Radiologist/physicians from private sector would be encouraged to provide voluntary services at public health facilities where government sector practitioners are not available or inadequate.
- Pregnant women would be given Mother and Child Protection Cards and safe motherhood booklet.

PMSMA- Stickers for Normal/ High risk Pregnancy

- One of the critical components of the Abhiyan is identification and follow up of high risk pregnancies. A sticker indicating the condition and risk factor of the pregnant women would be added onto MCP card for each visit:
- Green Sticker- for women with no risk factor detected
- Red Sticker – for women with high risk pregnancy
- A National Portal for PMSMA and a Mobile application have been developed to facilitate the engagement of private/ voluntary sector.
- 'IPledgeFor9' Achievers Awards have been devised to celebrate individual and team achievements and acknowledge voluntary contributions for PMSMA in states and districts across India.

Rashtriya Kishor Swasthya Karyakram (RKSK)

The Ministry of Health and Family welfare launched Rashtriya Kishor Swasthya Karyakram was launched on Jan 2014 for adolescents, in the age group of 10-19 years.

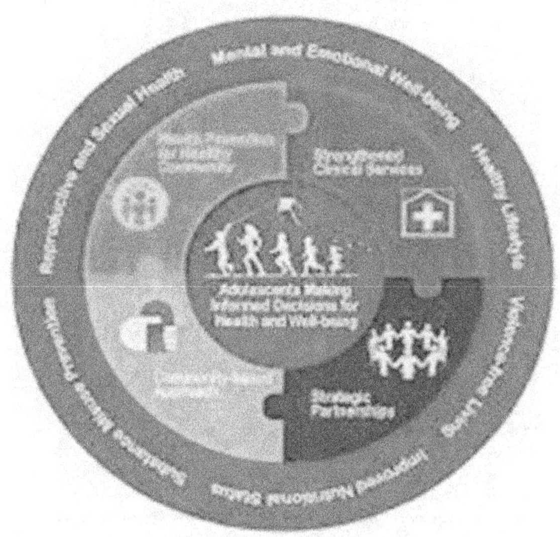

Figure 6: RKSK program components

The target of the program is

- **Improve their Nutrition**
- **Improve sexual and Reproductive Health**
- **Enhance Mental Health**
- **Prevent injuries and violence**
- **Prevent substance abuse**

Newer Initiatives (Saathiya Resource kit)

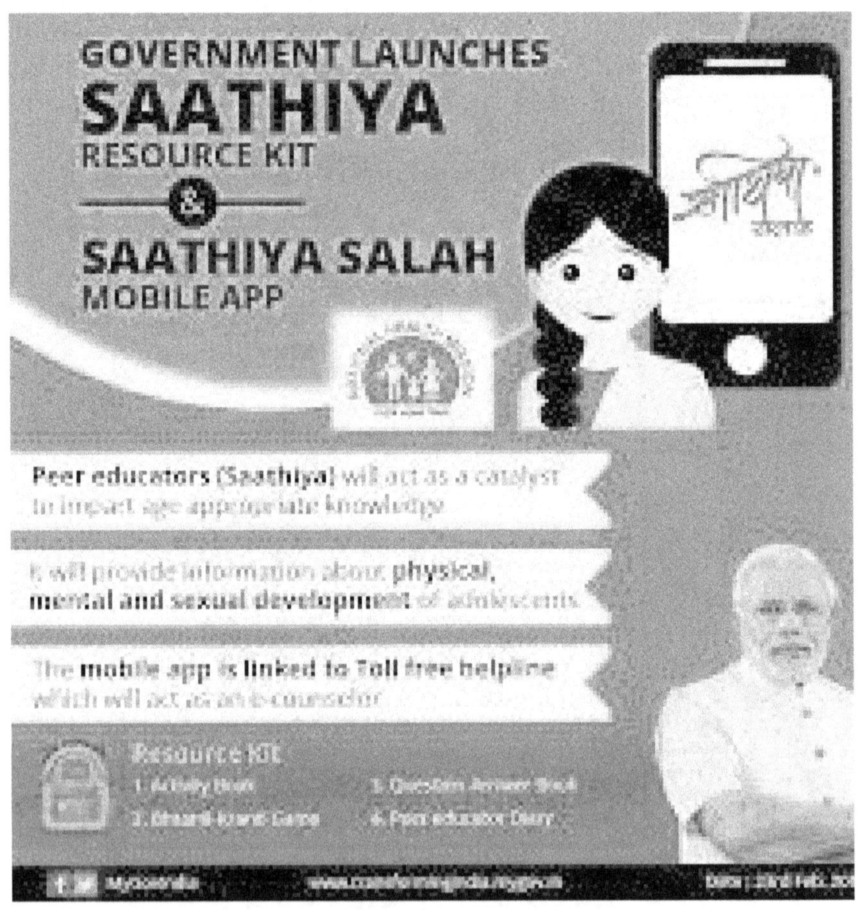

Figure 7: Saathiya Resource Kit- Mobile App

- Shri C.K Mishra, Secretary, Health and family welfare launched the SAATHIYA Resource Kit including Saathiya Salah Mobile App for adolescents.
- As part of the Rashtriya Kishor Swasthya Karyakaram (RKSK) program, one of the key interventions underthe programme is introduction of the Peer Educators(Saathiyas) who act as a catalyst for generating demand for the adolescent health issues to their peer groups.
- The peer educators will also play short films at their group meetings. The games and the activity books will bring about discussion and resolove around adolescent queries.

Training ASHAs & ANMs

- "Prevention of Post-Partum Hemorrhage (PPH) through Community based advance distribution of Misoprostol" by ASHAs/ANMs has been launched for high home delivery districts.
- Operational Guidelines and Reference Manual have beendisseminated to the States.
- However, during the counselling sessions with the pregnant women conducted by ASHAs and ANMs, emphasis is laid on the need to register for ANC and delivery at institutions

Village Health and Nutrition Days (VHNDs)

- **Monthly Village Health and Nutrition Days (VHNDs) is an outreach activity at Anganwadi centers for provision of maternal and childcare including nutrition in convergence with the ICDS.**
- **Village Health and Nutrition Days proposed to be organized once in a month at each Anganwadi Centre.**
- **ANM, Anganwadi Worker and ASHA will ensure their presence on Saturday (as per schedule) and will coordinate to make this activity at village level as an effective intervention**

Maternal Health Kit

- Maternal Health Tool Kit has been developed as a ready reckoner/handbook for programme managers to plan, implement and monitor services at health facilities.

- It focuses on the Delivery Points, which includes setting up with adequate physical infrastructure, ensuring

- logistics & supplies and recording/reporting & monitoring systems with the objective of providing good quality comprehensive RMNCH services.

Pre-Service Education- Nursing Midwifery cadre

Five National Nodal Centre (NNC) are established for Pre-Service Education for strengthening Nursing Midwifery Cadre

- College of Nursing, Vadodara.
- Kasturba Nursing College, Sewagram, Wardha.
- Regional College of Nursing, Guwahati.
- College of Nursing, Kanpur; and College of Nursing MMC, Chennai have been strengthened Achieving above 70% of performance standards, around 43% of the targeted ANM & GNM Nursing institutions in the high focus States have fully equipped mini-skill labs. 85% of these institutions have library and around 89%have IT labs.
- Capacity building of 700 nursing faculties in the country through customized 6 Week Training has been conducted and 6 days training of 250 nursing faculties also have been conducted at National Skills lab "Daksh".

Delivery Points

- More than 50 deliveries per month is conducted in health care center which is considered as delivery point.
- More than 20,000 'Delivery Points' have been identified across the country based on performance.

- Delivery Points will ensure assured services 24x7 hours of Mother and child care like, ANC, intrapartum, postnatal, Newborn and child care including family planning services.
- 24x7 PHCs and FRUs Doctors and staff Nurses will be trained for PPIUCD (Postpartum Intrauterine contraceptive Devices)

Capacity Building

- More than 50 deliveries per month is conducted in health care centre which is considered as delivery point.
- More than 20,000 'Delivery Points' have been identified across the country based on performance.
- Delivery Points will ensure assured services 24x7 hours of Mother and child care like, ANC, intrapartum, postnatal, Newborn and child care including family planning services.
- 24x7 PHCs and FRUs Doctors and staff Nurses will be trained for PPIUCD (Postpartum Intrauterine contraceptive Devices)

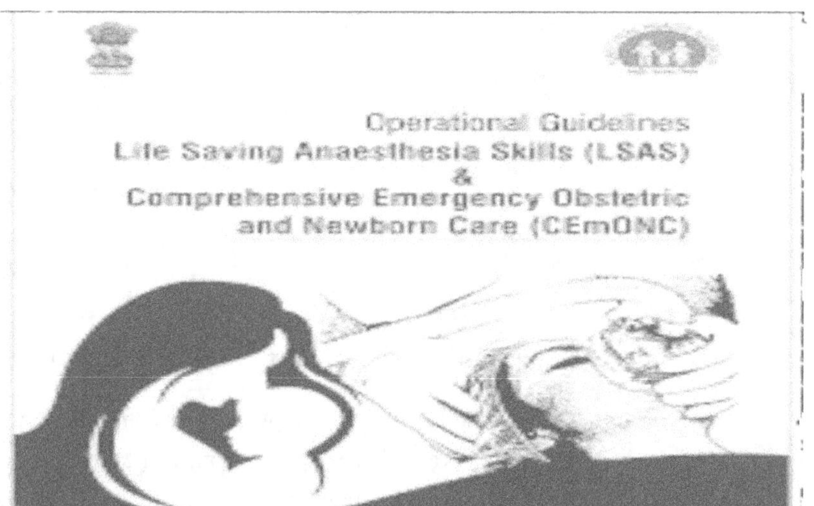

Figure 8: Operational guidelines manual-LSAS & CEmONC

Skill Labs

- Setting up of Skill Labs has been done with earmarked skill stations for different training programmes to strengthen the quality of capacity building of different cadres of service providers in the States.

- Guidelines and training modules of skill labs have been disseminated to the States.

- Five National Skills labs are now operational for conducting training of trainers.

- Skill labs have been established at different states such as Gujarat, Hayana, Maharashtra, MP, West Bengal, Odisha, Tamil Nadu and Karnataka.

- 1900 health personnel have been trained at the skill labs till date

Mother Child Tracking System (MCTS)

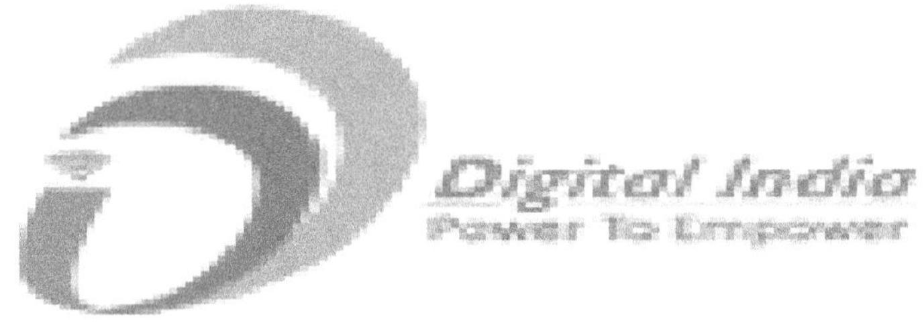

Figure 9: Mother Child Tracking System by Digital India

- Mother and Child Tracking System (MCTS) is an initiative of Health & Family Welfare to leverage information technology for ensuring delivery of full spectrum of health care and immunization services to pregnant women and children up to the age of 5 years.

- This Web Enabled Mother and Child Tracking System (MCTS) is being implemented to register and track every pregnant woman, neonate, infant and child by name for quality ANC, INC, PNC, FP, Immunisation services.

- It facilitâtes and monitors service delivery and also establishes a two way communication between the service providers and beneficiaries

Dakshata guidelines (New guidelines)

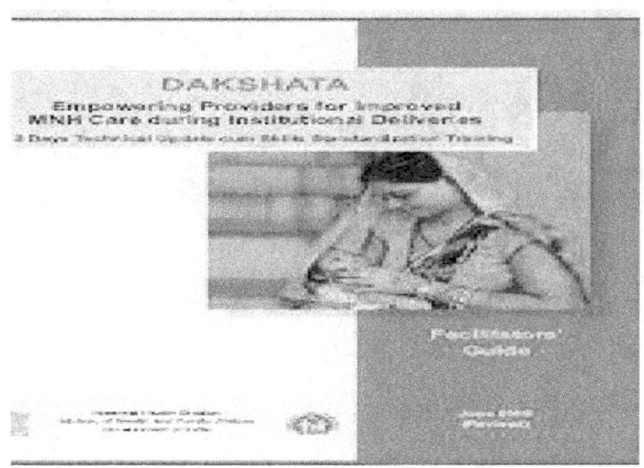

Figure 10: Dakshata guidelines (New guidelines) – Practice guidelines for intrapartum care

Dakshata guidelines for strengthening intra-partum care.

The main objectives of Dakshata are

---

1. **To strengthen the competency of providers of the labour room.**
2. **To implement evidence based clinical practices.**
3. **To improve the essential supplies and commodities in labour room**
4. **To improve recording, reporting and utilization of data**
5. **Implementation of MNH Tool Kit at the delivery points**

Checklist 1: Before Birth-Safe Childbirth Checklist (SCC)

Explain to call for help if there is:

- Bleeding
- Severe abdominal pain
- Difficulty in breathing
- Severe headache or blurred vision
- Urge to push
- Can't empty bladder every 2 hours
- NO OXYTOCIN/ other uterotonics for unnecessary induction/augmentation of labour
- Encouraged a birth companion to be present during labour at birth and till discharge-
  Yes/ No

Checklist 2: Just Before and During Birth (or C- Section)

a. **AMTSL- Ini. Oxytocin 10 units IM given withih ine minute of birth of the baby?**
   A. Yes
   B. No

b. **Breast feeding initiated in first half-an-hour of birth of the baby?**
   A. A.Yes
   B. B.No

(AMTSL- Active Management of Third stage of Labour)

Checklist 3: Soon after Birth (within 1 hour)

a. Started breastfeeding. Explain colostrum feeding is important for the baby- Yes/No
b. Started skin to skin contact (if mother and baby well) and KMC in pre- term and low-birth weight babies – Yes/No

Explain Checklist 4: Before Discharge

Danger Signs:

Mother has any of:

- Excessive bleeding
- Severe abdominal pain
- Severe headache or visual disturbances
- Breathing difficulties
- Fever or chills
- Difficulty emptying bladder
- Foul smelling vaginal discharge

The danger signs and confirm mother/ companion will call for help if danger signs present.

The Millennium development goals (2000-15) had listed one of the targets of reducing maternal mortality ratio (MMR) by three quarters from 1990 to 2015 (reducing the MMR from 560 in 1990 to 139 in 2015). the year 2015, the Sustainable Development Goal (SDG) target list has the target of decreasing MMR to 70 deaths per 1,00,000 live births by the year 2030. The available MMR data shows that maternal mortality in India varies significantly between States (Kerala's MMR=46; Assam's 237). These regional disparities must be addressed by implementing programs that improve the coverage of essential maternal health and strengthening health care infrastructure. While maternal health schemes are playing an important role in reducing maternal mortality, it is crucial that society at large plays a role. There should be an end to gender discriminatory practices which deter women from accessing reproductive and sexual heaths services. Child marriage and domestic violence are the evils of the society need to tackle and put to an end. Girl child education should be must for the women empowerment.

REFERENCE:

1. Deepak Sharma et.al.Health schemes for improving maternal health in India, Available from URL: http://gmch.gov.in
2. Maternal health. Available from URL: http://unicef.in/Whatwedo/1/Maternal-Health
3. Maternal mortality ratio. Available from URL: http://niti.gov.in/content/maternalmortality-ratio-mmr-100000-live-births.
4. Pradhan MantriMatruVandanaYojana. Maternal mortality ratio. Available from URL: http://niti.gov.in/content/maternalmortality-ratio-mmr-100000-live-births.
5. Janani Suraksha Yojana (JSY). https://www.nhp.gov.in/janani-suraksha-yojana-jsy-_pg
6. Janani Shishu Suraksha Karyakaram. URL: http://nhp.gov.in/jananishishu-suraksha-karyakaram-jssk_pg.
7. Sustainable development goals. Available from URL: http://www.undp.org/content/undp/en/home/sustainable-developmentgoals.html.
8. 8.Dakshata. Available from URL: http://nhm.gov.in/nrhm-components/rmnch-a/maternalhealth/dakshata/dakshata-3-days-training.html#.

3. MATERNAL MORTALTY

Each year in India, roughly 28 million women experience pregnancy and 26 million have a live birth, of these, an estimated 67,000 maternal deaths and one million newborn deaths occur each year. In addition, millions more women and newborns suffer pregnancy and childbirth related ill-health. Thus, pregnancy-related mortality and morbidity continues to have a huge impact on the lives of Indian women and their newborns.

MMR: According to WHO maternal mortality defined as the death of a woman while pregnant or within 42 days of termination of pregnancy

MMR ratio:

$$MMR = \frac{\text{Total no of female deaths due to complications of pregnancy, childbirth or within 42 days of delivery from puerperal causes in an area during a giver year MMR}}{\text{Total no.of live births in the same area and year}} \times \frac{1000}{(or) \ 100,000}$$

Maternal Mortality rate- - Worldwide

- Maternal mortality is unacceptably high. About 295 000 women died during and following pregnancy and childbirth in 2017. The vast majority of these deaths (94%) occurred in low- resource settings, and most could have been prevented.
- Sub-Saharan Africa and Southern Asia accounted for approximately 86% (254 000) of the estimated global maternal deaths in 2017.

- Sub-Saharan Africa alone accounted for roughly two-thirds (196 000) of maternal deaths, while Southern Asia accounted for nearly one-fifth (58 000).

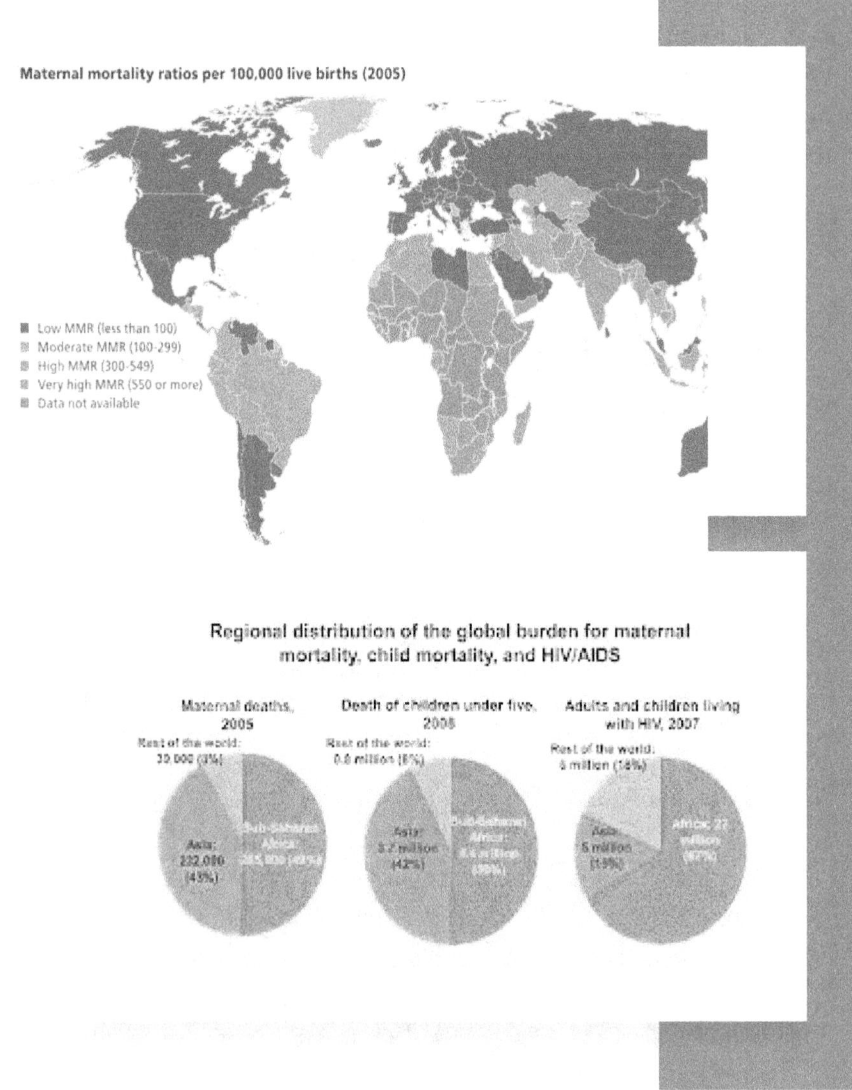

Figure 11: Worldwide Maternal Mortality Rate (MMR)

Global decline in maternal mortality rate

- At the same time, between 2000 and 2017, Southern Asia achieved the greatest overall reduction in MMR: a decline of nearly 60% (from an MMR of 384 down to 157).

- Despite its very high MMR in 2017, sub-Saharan Africa as a sub-region also achieved a substantial reduction in MMR of nearly 40% since 2000.

- Additionally, four other sub- regions roughly halved their MMRs during this period: Central Asia, Eastern Asia, Europe, and Northern Africa.

- Overall, the maternal mortality ratio (MMR) in less-developed countries declined by just under 50%.

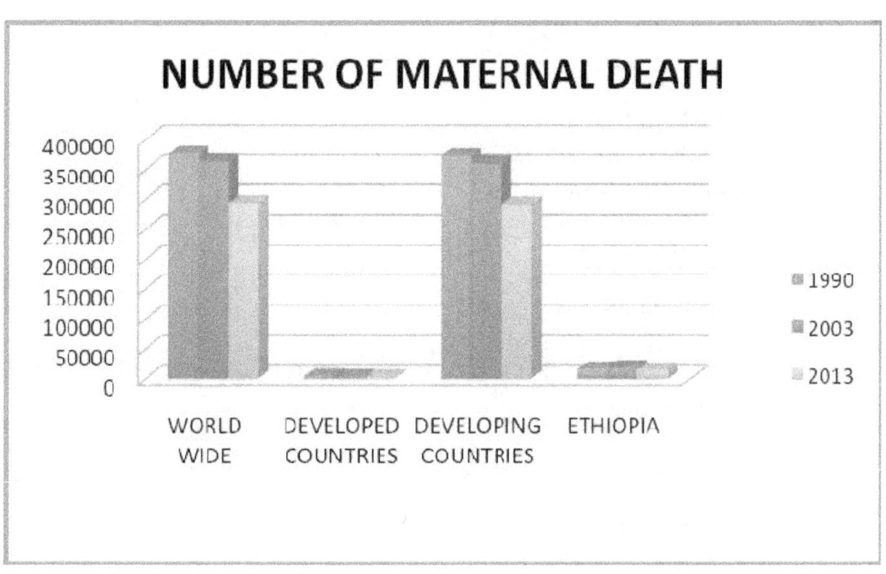

Figure 12: Global Decline in Maternal Death - (1990 – 2013)

- The high number of maternal deaths in some areas of the world reflects inequalities in access to quality health services and highlights the gap between rich and poor.

- The MMR in low-income countries in 2017 is 462 per 100 000 live births versus 11 per 100 000 live births in high income countries.

- 99% of all maternal deaths occur in the developing countries

- Sub Saharan Africa and Southern Asian countries account for most maternal deaths.

Causes of MMR- Worldwide

- **Severe bleeding (25%)**
- **Infection (15%)**
- **Eclampsia (12%)**
- **Obstructed labour (8%)**
- **Unsafe abortion (13%)**

- **Other direct causes (8%)**

- **Indirect causes (20%)**

    a. **Indirect causes including anaemia, malaria, heart diseases.**

    b. **Other direct causes including ectopic pregnancy, embolism, aesthesia related.**

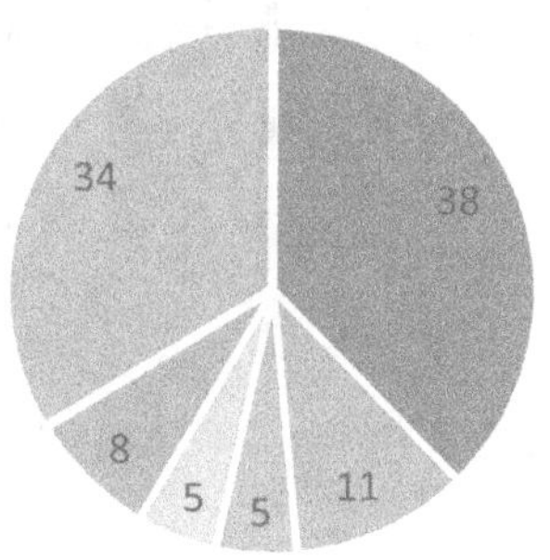

Figure 13: Causes of MMR in India

Causes of MMR in India

Haemorrhage (38%)

Sepsis (11%)

Hypertensive Disorders (5%)

Obstructed labour (5%)

Abortion (8%)

Other Conditions (34%)

The common reasons Maternal Death and preventive Strategies:

Haemorrhage

- **Severe Bleeding:** After birth can kill a healthy woman within hours if she is unattended. Injecting oxytocin immediately after childbirth effectively reduces the risk of bleeding.

- Plasma expanders (Plasma Protein) - Treatment of circulatory Shock

- Referral to an equipped facility must be available to woman with PPH
- NASG – Non-Pneumatic antishock Garment. It stabilizes a woman in shock and haemorrhage, and this can save a woman's life

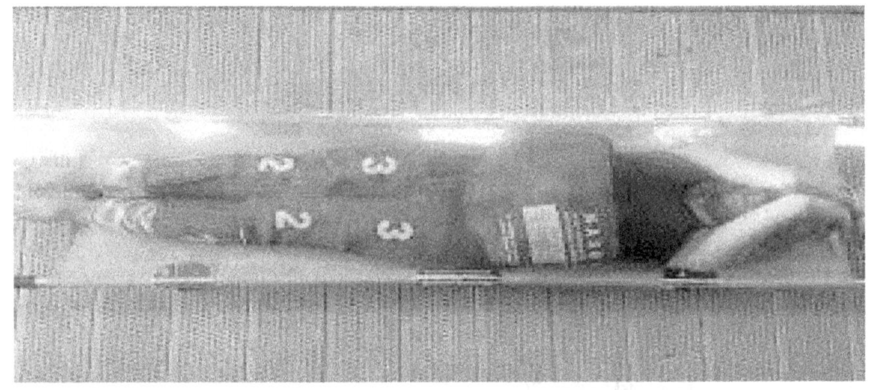

Figure 14: NASG – Non-Pneumatic Antishock Garment

Obstructed labour:

- Monitoring Partograph during labour for early identification of any deviation from normal progress.

- Delivery of those woman with obstructed labour must be in facility offering trained doctors and well-equipped operating rooms.

Pre- Eclampsia:

Unsafe Abortion:

- The WHO estimates that almost half a million woman in developing countries die in pregnancy and childbirth every year. Unsafe abortion is responsible for 100-400/100,000 deaths which accounts for 25-50% of all maternal deaths. Whereas in safe abortion the maternal deaths are estimated 6/200,000.
- Even when woman survive the procedure, there are numerous possible physical complications includes incomplete abortion, Pelvic Infection, hemorrhage, Shock, and secondary sterility. Also, enormous costs to the health care system for treating abortion complications.
- Safe, legal services for terminating unwanted pregnancies be offered as an integral part of national primary health care systems.

Rupture of Uterus:

It is caused by Mismanagement during labour in case of Previous LSCS-VBAC, Myomectomy, Uterine Perforation (D&C, Forceps delivery) and Oxytocin drugs. It can be prevented by following Operational Guidelines manual & Dakshata Guidelines during intrapartum care.

Cardiac Arrest:

- **Obstetric causes include haemorrhage, eclampsia, and amniotic fluid embolism.**

- **Non- obstetric causes are sepsis, pulmonary embolism, pre-existing cardiovascular diseases and stroke.**

- **Iatrogenic causes include aesthetic complications during delivery or testing.**

Obstetric CPR: When a woman is found to be unresponsive and not breathing properly:

- Call for help

- One person should immediately start high-quality CPR at a rate of 30 compressions to 2 breaths

- One person should manage her airway (provide ventilation with bag-valve mask and intubation)

- And someone should apply manual left uterine displacement to help ensure proper blood flow to the heart. (Push the women's uterus towards left side)

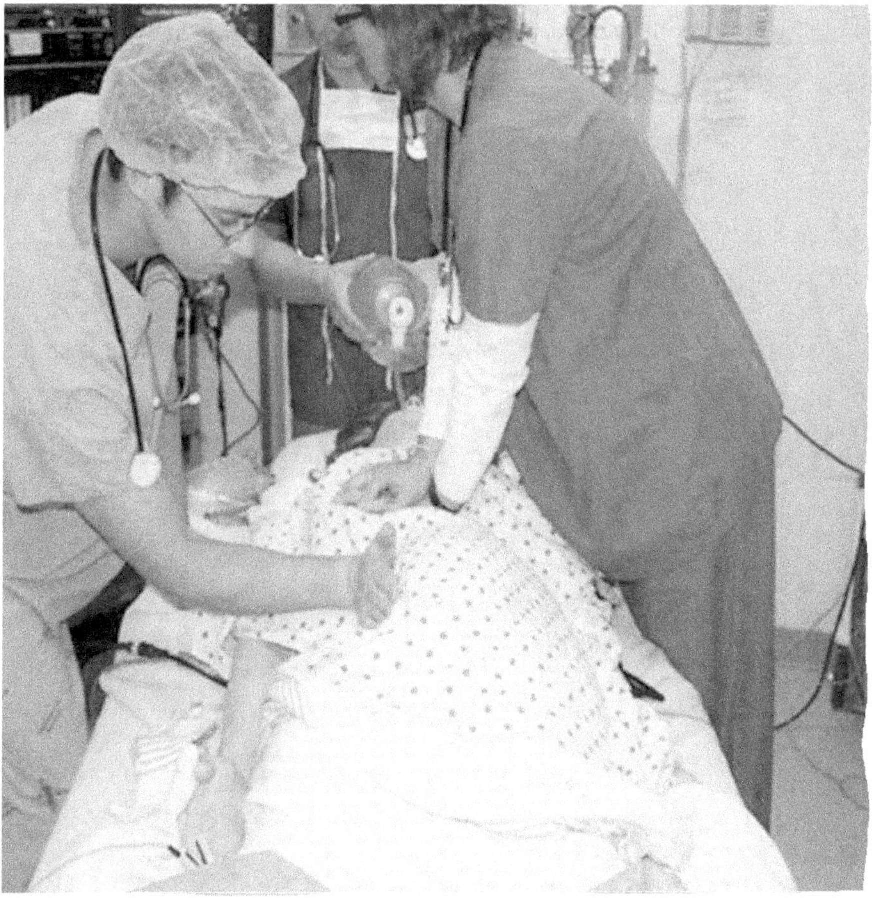

Figure 15: Obstetric CPR

WHO Response -MMR

World Health Organization

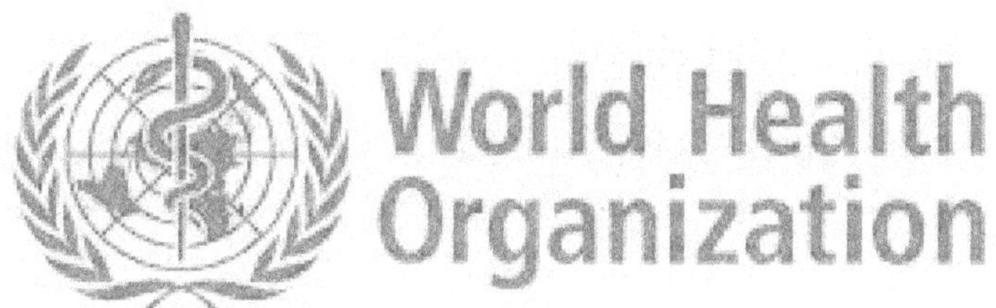

- Addressing inequalities in access to and quality of reproductive, maternal, and newborn health care services.

- Ensuring universal health coverage for comprehensive reproductive, maternal, and newborn health care.

- Addressing all causes of maternal mortality, reproductive and maternal morbidities, and related disabilities.

- Strengthening health systems to collect high quality data in order to respond to the needs and priorities of women and girls.

- Addressing inequalities in access to and quality of reproductive, maternal, and newborn health care services.

- Ensuring universal health coverage for comprehensive reproductive, maternal, and newborn health care.

- Addressing all causes of maternal mortality, reproductive and maternal morbidities, and related disabilities;

- Strengthening health systems to collect high quality data in order to respond to the needs and priorities of women and girls.

The sustainable developmental goals:

- **In the context of the Sustainable Development Goals (SDG), countries have united behind a new target to accelerate the decline of maternal mortality by 2030.**

- **SDG 3 includes an ambitious target:**

"Reducing the global MMR to less than 70 per 100,000 births, with no country having a maternal mortality rate of more than twice the global average".

Effective Strategies to reduce MMR in India:

- Prenatal care includes nutritional supplements and obstetrical examination

- Targeting woman suffering from toxaemia, bleeding, and infections

- Local ambulances with life support equipment and maternity waiting houses.

- Referral centres should be capable of providing sterile conditions and blood transfusions

- Referrals by trained birth attendants

Roles and responsibly of a community health Nurse:

- To improve quality of MCH care at the rural community level (which includes proper history taking, palpation, blood pressure and foetal heart rate screening, risk factor screening and referral)

- To improve the quality of care at the primary health care level (emergency care and proper referral).

- Attention should be directed to delivery practices and facilities, which accounts for most of the Maternal mortality. (Clean and well-equipped labour room).

- High-risk risk mothers should be housed in Maternity waiting homes located near Hospitals.

- To give attention to care during labour and delivery, which is the most critical period of complications.

- **Antenatal care with risk referral**
- **Health education about Maternal Health Schemes**
- **Encourage small family norms among postnatal mothers**
- **Create awareness about family planning methods**
- **Practice labour room protocols**
- **Emphasis legal, medical abortion**
- **No augmentation of labour unnecessarily**
- **Faculty should incorporate WHO/ Govt of India guidelines while demonstrating midwifery procedures to UG/PG-OBG students.**

Maternal Mortality Ratio (MMR) in India was exceptionally high in 1990 with 556 women dying during childbirth per hundred thousand live births. Approximately, 1.38 lakh women were dying every year on account of complications related to pregnancy and childbirth. The global MMR at the time was much lower at 385. There has, however, been an accelerated decline in MMR in India. MMR in the country has declined to 167 (2011-13) against a global MMR of 216 (2015). The maternal mortality ratio (MMR) between 2016 and 2018 dripped to 113 in India, almost 100 deaths lesser than in 2007- 2008 period.

Reference:

1. Trends in maternal mortality: 2000 to 2017: estimates by WHO, UNICEF, UNFPA, World Bank Group and the United Nations Population Division. Geneva: World Health Organization; 2019.

2. (2) Ganchimeg T, Ota E, Morisaki N, et al. Pregnancy and childbirth outcomes among adolescent mothers: a World Health Organization multicountry study. BJOG 2014;121 Suppl 1:40–8.

3. (3) Althabe F, Moore JL, Gibbons L, et al. Adverse maternal and perinatal outcomes in adolescent pregnancies: The Global Network's Maternal Newborn Health Registry study. Reprod Health 2015;12 Suppl 2:S8.

4. (4) Say L, Chou D, Gemmill A, Tunçalp Ö, Moller AB, Daniels JD, et al. Global Causes of Maternal Death: A WHO Systematic Analysis. Lancet Global Health. 2014;2(6): e323-e333.

5. (5) World Health Organization and United Nations Children's Fund. WHO/UNICEF joint database on SDG 3.1.2 Skilled Attendance at Birth. Available at: https://unstats.un.org/sdgs/indicators/database/

6. (6) Strategies towards ending preventable maternal mortality (EPMM).Geneva: World Health Organization; 2015.

4. ETHICS AND SIADARDS OF MIDWIFERY

This Code of Ethics and Standards of Professional Conduct for Nurses and Midwives applies to the nurses and midwives registered in all the state Nursing councils in India. Also, this guidelines provides a framework for professional accountability and responsibility of nursing and midwifery practices as per the regulations of International confederation of midwives (ICM) to improve the standards of provided to women, newborns, and families throughout the world through education and appropriate utilization of professional midwife. This code acknowledge woman as persons with human rights, seeks justice for all people and equity in access to health care, and is based on mutual relationships of respect.

The Code contains a series of statements that taken together promotes good nursing and midwifery practice. These statements put the interests of patients and service users first, are safe and effective, and promotes trust through professionalism. They serve as a reference guide for ethical decisions that arise during practice and inform society about the ethical obligations and professional conduct that is expected from nurses and midwives. The Code also specifies the ethical obligations expected from management, educators, and researchers over and above the generic statements.

Ethical obligations for nurse/midwifery managers:

This section covers the role and responsibilities of nursing and midwifery managers in ensuring that the principles stated in this document are adhered to. Individual practitioners are responsible for their actions and obliged to adhere to the principles of the Code of ethics and Standards of Professional Conduct however nursing and midwifery management also play a strategic role in the actual fulfilment of these obligations.

Management must assist and support nurses and midwives to integrate high ethical standards of care and core values in everyday practice. One of the primary aims is to protect patient interests and safety and ensure the delivery of high-quality care. Management should provide opportunities for nurses and midwives to reach their professional competence. These range from ensuring correct staffing levels in order to provide space whereby nurses and midwives can attend for in-house training, lobby and/or organize professional development activities based on specific needs assessment. They must also work towards developing and maintaining an organizational culture which strives towards the upholding ethical standards and continuous professional development.

Managers have a responsibility to take care of their staff and provide the necessary support and guidance to tackle ethical dilemmas. They have a responsibility towards empowering staff nurses and midwives to act as advocates to minimize the risk of moral distress caused by feelings of powerlessness with regards to patient safety and well-being. They should encourage and assist in the development and attendance of ethical training.

The manager position is often faced with a barrage of decisions which requires substantial ethical fortitude from the individual to maintain and ensure that the safety and quality of care is not compromised. This is achieved if the managers themselves ensure that they keep abreast with ethical and leadership management throughout their position. This can also be achieved through individual or group reflective practice. The aim of these updates is to provide managers with a chance to explore various viewpoints and develop further their moral decision-making skills.

Ethical obligations for nurse/midwifery Educators:

The ethical obligations of educators cannot be undermined. Nursing and midwifery educators, in particular those in charge of undergraduate training, are responsible to educate students on the values, principles and standards presented in this document so that from an early stage they appreciate the ethical implications that the profession holds. Educators are encouraged to create an environment that embraces and supports on-going professional growth and competence. They should foster an inquisitive approach to education to instill a culture of innovation and creativity within their students. This will help students question the status quo and adopt evidence-based practice to improve and provide quality care. This entails that the educators themselves also engage in professional lifelong learning.

Nursing and midwifery educators can enhance professional integrity with the students. This can be achieved by encouraging and modelling professional behaviors that demonstrate honesty, respect for self and others, accountability, and self-growth. There should be a push towards teamwork and teambuilding throughout the training to increase the confidence in colleagues and in their patients. They have a responsibility to empower students to safeguard the patient, family, and society when they are endangered by health care professionals. Students should also be taught the importance of formulating and taking decisions based on ethical principles.

Students are the future generations of the professions. Educators are responsible to sensitise students to the importance of setting up of professional standards and research which will help in the advancement of the nursing and midwifery profession. They are also responsible to ensure that the quality of nursing and midwifery training is continually reviewed and revised to reflect latest guidelines and standards.

Ethical obligations for nurse/midwifery Researchers:

This section is intended for nurses and midwives who are:

- **Lead researchers of research projects.**

- **Involved in research as research assistants such as collecting or inputting data for research team.**

- **Responsible for patients participating in research.**

- **Involved in interpreting and using research as a basis for their practice; and**

- **Educators responsible for teaching and supervising research projects.**

Research helps to guide practice and improve the health and wellbeing of patients through the application of evidence-based practice. This document stipulates that nurses and midwives have a commitment to research through evidence-based practice is elicited. Nurses and midwives must ensure that the following ethical obligations are adhered to prior to conducting the research.

The ethical principles that govern nurses and midwives practice also apply to ethical principles for research. These include the respect of person, justice, and beneficence. These ethical considerations that should be kept in mind by nursing and midwifery researchers when conducting or participating in research. These considerations include obtaining permission from the relevant research ethics committee, informed consent, confidentiality, and vulnerability.

The concerned research ethics committee must approve the research protocol. The role of research ethics committees is to scrutinize the protocol to ensure that the proposed research protects the rights and safety of the study participants. This is particularly important since some participants in nursing and midwifery research are potentially vulnerable and may have an increased risk of incurring additional harm. Such participants include children, certain groups of adults such as unconscious patients, terminally ill, some elderly people and those with mental health needs. These groups should only be chosen if they are to benefit from the knowledge, practices or interventions that result from the research findings.

Another important consideration is informed consent. Researchers must ensure that participants are provided with adequate information about the study aim, methodology, possible conflict of interest, funding, inconveniences and demands on them, anticipated benefits, and potential risks of the study prior to seeking the participants' potential voluntary informed consent. Participants need to be informed about their right to refuse or withdraw from the study at any time if they change their mind. They should also be informed that irrelevant of their reply to their care will not be compromised in anyway.

The same ethical considerations must be upheld when patient records are used in research. In addition to the ethical obligations, the researchers must also ensure that they adhere to the institutional policy regarding medical records, and the relevant data protection legislation.
Nurses and midwives participating in clinical trials need to be aware of the potential risks and benefits of patients to ensure that participants are always protected. Nurses and midwives must also be aware that clinical trials are regulated by the Clinical Trial Regulations in India.

Respect towards colleagues:

Ethical Principles

As members of the professions, nurses and midwives must:

1. Respect knowledge, experience, expertise, and insights of other colleagues.

2. Respect colleagues irrespective of age, nationality, gender, religious beliefs, sexual orientation, and political inclination and work with them in a professional, collaborative and co-operative manner within the scope of practice.

3. Take every opportunity to pass on their skills and knowledge to colleagues, junior staff and students and be responsible for the professional behavior of those under their charge.

4. Be bound to report any willful malpractice and / or professional incompetence to the appropriate authorities as well as any circumstance where it appears that the health and safety of colleagues is at risk and may compromise standards of good practice and care.

5. Maintain a safe working environment, which does not pose any additional risk to colleagues.

6. Recognize their role in delegating care appropriately and in providing the necessary supervision.

Standards of Professional Conduct:

Nurses and midwives must

- Ask for advice and assistance from colleagues especially when care may be compromised by lack of knowledge or skill.

- Work together to resolve any differences in a constructive way.

- Refrain from passing criticism or malicious comments about colleagues which may undermine the patient's trust in them.

- Co-operate with other members of the health care team for the optimal delivery of care; nurses and midwives should accept and value the diversity of co-workers and acknowledge the need for non-discriminatory interpersonal and interprofessional relationships.

- Communicate clearly, effectively, respectfully, and promptly with other colleagues in particular handing over.

- Ensure appropriate communication (both verbal and written) within a legal and ethical framework.

Maintaining public trust and confidence:

Ethical Principles

As members of the professions, nurses and midwives must

- Act lawfully whether those laws relate to the professional practice or personal life.

- Recognize their responsibility to clarify, secure, and sustain ethical nursing and midwifery conduct.

- Retain a commitment for patient wellbeing in all professional settings, including education, research, and administration.

- Promote patient safety and wellbeing in all circumstances.

- Share with other citizens the responsibility for initiating and supporting actions designed to maintain and improve the health and social needs of the public.

- Ensure that their professional status is not used in the promotion of commercial products or services. Nurses and midwives shall also ensure that their professional judgement is not influenced by any commercial consideration.

- Advocate for equity and social justice in resource allocation, access to health care and other social and economic services.

- Ensure economical effectiveness and appropriate management of healthcare resources based on evidence-based practice.

Standards of professional conduct:

Nurses and midwives must

- Bear an obligation to behave in such a way as to maintain public trust and confidence in nurses and midwives and the professions they always represent.

- Demonstrate a personal commitment to equality and diversity.

- Be kind and compassionate in their practice.

- Respect the property and resources belonging to patients, colleagues, and organizations.

- Document and report one's concerns according to established policies if the work environment is compromising the health and safety of the workers and patient.

- Report to their superiors or regulatory authority if they believe that the health, professional competence or conduct of a colleague will compromise public safety or bring the profession into disrepute.

- Ensure that any use of substances or medicines are not compromising nursing or midwifery practice.

- Participate in research in accordance with recognized guidelines.

- Ensure a professional image which projects competency, inspires confidence and communicates respect to patients/clients, co-workers, and the public.
- Maintain their personal health and well-being responsibly. Seek assistance and inform their superiors as appropriate if their health threatens the ability to practice safely.
- Do not misuse their professional position to promote or sell products or services for personal gain.
- Act in ways that cannot be interpreted as, or do not result in, their gaining personal benefit from their position in nursing or midwifery.
- Refrain from accepting gifts, favours or hospitality as it may compromise the professional relationship with the patient under one's care. Nurses and midwives are advised to refer to the document 'Professional Boundaries for Nurses and Midwives'.
- Refrain from accepting power of attorney responsibilities for patient under their care to make legal and financial decisions on their behalf.
- Do not engage in sexual, intimate behavior or a personal relationship with patients, their families and/or their significant others during their care.
- Actively participate in good clinical governance to ensure safe and optimal care.
- Use healthcare resources effectively at one's work setting.

Professional responsibilities of Nurse/Midwife:

- People and society trust nurses and midwives with their health and well-being. It is implicit that nurses and midwives reciprocate back by always acting legally and in an ethically correct way.
- Whenever a course of action will affect patients, their welfare must always be the uppermost priority whether the action is the result of management, the educational system or research.

- The conduct of research must conform to bioethical nursing /midwifery practice. When patients or their notes are to be used as teaching or assessing resources, they must be used with great sensitivity. Management must ensure that although its decisions often only affect patients in groups, it must at all times consider the impact of its decisions upon the In these contexts, the self-direction of patients takes on added importance. Above all, prior informed consent is required for participation in research or teaching, and all reasonable precautions should be taken to ensure that patients come to no harm.

- Working conditions should contribute to high standards of care and to professional satisfaction. Nurses and midwives should work towards securing and maintaining working conditions and environments that satisfy these inter-related goals.

- Nurses and midwives should consider how they can contribute to improving staffing levels, to obtain adequate supplies and equipment, to make the best use of available resources, and to maintain high standards of hygiene. Nurses and midwives should resist the introduction of roster or any other professional issues which may result in a lowering of standards of care. They should also strive to have the worth of their work appreciated and adequately remunerated.

- The close interaction with the patients, families and communities provides nurses and midwives with valuable knowledge of health needs within the society. Hence, nurses and midwives are well positioned to provide advice and support actions designed to address these health care needs.

- Nurses and midwives must ensure that their professional status is not used to advertise commercial products or services. They should, moreover, declare any financial or other interests in relevant organizations providing such goods or services, and ensure that their professional judgement is not influenced by any commercial considerations such as commission, and gifts.

- Nurses and midwives must advocate for accessible health care services to be provided when needed and considers and takes actions to address social injustice whenever it arises. Nurses and midwives should pay attention to the social determinants of health and ensure that patients are not discriminated or suffer social injustice because of their background or social status. Nurses and midwives can act individually or collectively to ensure that actions are being taken to reduce social inequalities to achieve health for all at policy level.
- Nurses and midwives must make best use of available resources to improve efficiency and reduce waste. Nurses and midwives must also make judicious use of supplies and use the right products to ensure cost-effective care.

Code of Ethics for Nurses in India:

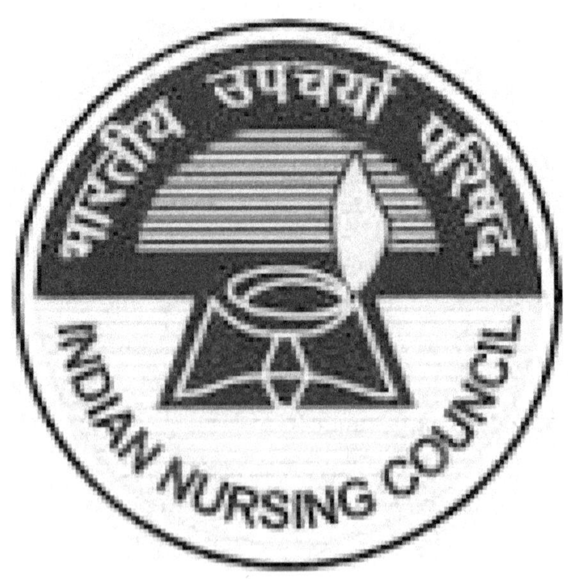

The nurse respects the uniqueness of individual in provision of care
Nurse

1.1 Provides care of individuals without consideration of caste, creed, religion,
culture, ethnicity, gender, socio-economic and political status, personal attributes,
or any other grounds
1.2 Individualizes the care considering the beliefs, values, and cultural sensitivities
1.3 Appreciates the place of individual in the family and community and facilitates
participation of significant others in the care.
1.4 Develops and promotes trustful relationship with individual(s)
1.5 Recognizes uniqueness of response of individuals to interventions and adapts
Accordingly

---

2. The nurse respects the rights of individuals as partner in care and help in making informed choices
Nurse

2.1 Appreciates individual's right to make decisions about their care and therefore gives adequate and accurate information for enabling them to make informed choices
2.2 Respects the decisions made by individual(s) regarding their care
2.3 Protects public from misinformation and misinterpretations
2.4 Advocates special provision to protect vulnerable individuals/groups.

3.The nurse respects individual's right to privacy, maintains confidentiality, and shares information judiciously
Nurse

3.1 **Respects the individual's right to privacy of their personal information**
3.2 Maintains confidentiality of privileged information except in life threatening
   situations and uses discretion in sharing information.
3.3 Takes informed consent and maintains anonymity when information is required
   for quality assurance/ academic/legal reasons
3.4 Limits the access to all personal records written and computerized to authorized
persons only.

---

4. Nurse maintains competence in order to render Quality Nursing Care
Nurse

4.1 Nursing care must be provided only by registered nurse
4.2 Nurse strives to maintain quality nursing care and upholds the standards of care
4.3 Nurse values continuing education, initiates and utilizes all opportunities for self development.
4.4 Nurses values research as a means of development of nursing profession and participates in nursing research adhering to ethical principles.

---

5. The nurse if obliged to practice within the framework of ethical, professional and legal boundaries
Nurse

5.1 Adheres to code of ethics and code of professional conduct for nurses in India
developed by Indian Nursing Council
5.2 Familiarizes with relevant laws and practices in accordance with the law of the
State

---

6. Nurse is obliged to work harmoniously with members of the health team
Nurse

6.1 Appreciates the team efforts in rendering care
6.2 Cooperates, coordinates, and collaborates with members of the health team to meet
the needs of people

---

7. Nurse commits to reciprocate the trust invested in nursing profession by society
Nurse

7.1 Demonstrates personal etiquettes in all dealings
7.2 Demonstrates professional attributes in all dealings

Code of Professional Conduct for Nurses in India

1. Professional Responsibility and accountability
Nurse

1.1 Appreciates sense of self-worth and nurtures it

1.2 Maintains standards of personal conduct reflecting credit upon the profession

1.3 Carries out responsibilities within the framework of the professional boundaries

1.4 Is accountable for maintaining practice standards set by Indian Nursing Council

1.5 Is accountable for own decisions and actions

1.6 Is compassionate

1.7 Is responsible for continuous improvement of current practices

1.8 Provides adequate information to individuals that allows them informed choices

1.9 Practices healthful behaviour

2. Nursing Practice
Nurse

2.1 Provides care in accordance with set standards of practice

2.2 Treats all individuals and families with human dignity in providing physical, psychological, emotional, social and spiritual aspects of care

2.3 Respects individuals and families in the context of traditional and cultural practices, promoting healthy practices and discouraging harmful practices

2.4 Presents realistic picture truthfully in all situations for facilitating autonomous decision-making by individuals and families

2.5 Promotes participation of individuals and significant others in the care

2.6 Ensures safe practice

2.7 Consults, coordinates, collaborates, and follows up appropriately when individuals' care needs exceed the nurse's competence

3. Communication and Interpersonal Relationships
Nurse

3.1 Establishes and maintains effective interpersonal relationships with individuals,
families and communities
3.2 Upholds the dignity of team members and maintains effective interpersonal
relationship with them
3.3 Appreciates and nurtures professional role of team members
3.4 Cooperates with other health professional to meet the needs of the individuals,
families and communities

4. Valuing Human Being
Nurse

4.1 Takes appropriate action to protect individuals from harmful unethical practice
4.2 Considers relevant facts while taking conscience decisions in the best interest of
individuals
4.3 Encourages and supports individuals in their right to speak for themselves on
issues affecting their health and welfare
4.4 Respects and supports choices made by individuals

5. Management
Nurse

5.1 Ensures appropriate allocation and utilization of available resources
5.2 Participates in supervision and education of students and other formal care
providers
5.3 Uses judgment in relation to individual competence while accepting and delegating responsibility

5.4 Facilitates conductive work culture in order to achieve institutional objectives

5.5 Communicates effectively following appropriate channels of communication

5.6 Participates in performance appraisal

5.7 Participates in evaluation of nursing services

5.8 Participates in policy decisions, following the principle of equity and accessibility
of services

5.9 Works with individuals to identify their needs and sensitizes policy makers and
funding agencies for resource allocation

6. Professional Advancement
Nurse

6.1 Ensures the protection of the human rights while pursuing the advancement of
knowledge

6.2 Contributes to the development of nursing practice

6.3 Participates in determining and implementing quality care

6.4 Takes responsibility for updating own knowledge and competencies

6.5 Contributes to core of professional knowledge by conducting and participating in
research

The Code of Ethics

I. *Midwifery Relationships*

a. Midwives develop a partnership with individual women in which they share relevant information that leads to informed decision-making, consent to an evolving plan of care, and acceptance of responsibility for the outcomes of their choices.

b. Midwives support the right of women/families to participate actively in decisions about their care.

c. Midwives empower women/families to speak for themselves on issues affecting the health of women and families within their culture/society.

d. Midwives, together with women, work with policy and funding agencies to define women's needs for health services and to ensure that resources are fairly allocated considering priorities and availability.

e. Midwives support and sustain each other in their professional roles, and actively nurture their own and others' sense of self-worth.

f. Midwives respectfully work with other health professionals, consulting and referring as necessary when the woman's need for care exceeds the competencies of the midwife.

g. Midwives recognise the human interdependence within their field of practice and actively seek to resolve inherent conflicts.

h. Midwives have responsibilities to themselves as persons of moral worth, including duties of moral self-respect and the preservation of integrity.

II. *Practice of Midwifery*

a. Midwives provide care for women and childbearing families with respect for cultural diversity while also working to eliminate harmful practices within those same cultures.

b. Midwives encourage the minimum expectation that no woman or girl should be harmed by conception or childbearing.

c. Midwives use up-to-date, evidence-based professional knowledge to maintain competence in safe midwifery practices in all environments and cultures.

d. Midwives respond to the psychological, physical, emotional, and spiritual needs of women seeking health care, whatever their circumstances (non-discrimination).

e. Midwives act as effective role models of health promotion for women throughout their life cycle, for families and for other health professionals.

f. Midwives actively seek personal, intellectual, and professional growth throughout their midwifery career, integrating this growth into their practice.

III. *The Professional Responsibilities of Midwives*

a. Midwives hold in confidence client information in order to protect the right to privacy, and use judgment in sharing this information except when mandated by law.

b. Midwives are responsible for their decisions and actions, and are accountable for the related outcomes in their care of women.

c. Midwives may decide not to participate in activities for which they hold deep moral opposition: however, the emphasis on individual conscience should not deprive women of essential health services.

d. Midwives with conscientious objection to a given service request will refer the woman to another provider where such a service can be provided.

e. Midwives understand the adverse consequences that ethical and human rights violations have on the health of women and infants, and will work to eliminate these violations.

f. Midwives participate in the development and implementation of health policies that promote the health of all women and childbearing families.

IV. *Advancement of Midwifery Knowledge and Practice*

a. Midwives ensure that the advancement of midwifery knowledge is based on activities that protect the rights of women as persons.

b. Midwives develop and share midwifery knowledge through a variety of processes, such as peer review and research.

c. Midwives contribute to the formal education of midwifery students and on going education of midwives.

The code of ethics in midwifery practice addresses the ethical mandates in keeping standards of midwifery practices to promote the health and well- being of women and newborns within their families and communities. This care may encompass the reproductive cycle of the women from pre-pregnancy stage to menopause and to the end of life. These mandates include how midwives relate to others; how they practice midwifery; how they upload professional responsibilities and duties; and how they are to work to assure the integrity of the profession of midwifery.

Keywords

Accountability: being able to give an account of one's judgement, actions and omissions.

Adverse Event: an incident which resulted in or could have resulted in harm.

Advocate: the nurse or midwife should act and support the interest of the patient or client when she/he is unable to do so for himself/herself because of his/her limitations. In advocacy, nurses and midwives have primarily, to understand accurately the patient's wishes and needs.

Competence: the ability to practice safely and effectively fulfilling his/her professional responsibility within their scope of practice.

Co-workers: nurses/midwives, other health and non-health related workers and professionals.

Clinical Governance: a system through which health care organizations are accountable for continuously improving the quality of their services and safeguarding high standards of care by creating an environment in which excellence in clinical care will flourish.

Culturally Appropriate: practices that meet and respect cultural needs and differences.

Delegation: The transfer of a task or activity to a competent individual who is trained and certified to carry out that task or activity.

Evidence-Based Practice: health care decisions based on the best available evidence and clinical expertise.

Inaction: failure to act in a situation where action is required.

Integrity: upholding the values of the profession and the accepted standards of practice.

Omission: failure to act, especially when there is a moral or legal obligation to do.

Patient: a person who uses health and social care services. In some instances the terms 'client', 'mother' and 'individual' are used in place of the term patient depending on the context.

Personal Health: mental, physical, social and spiritual wellbeing of the nurse/midwife.

Reference

1. International confederation of midwives, Available in URL: https://www.international midwives.org
2. Code of Ethics for Nurses in India, Available in URL: https://www.tamilnadunursingcouncil.com
3. Code of conduct for nurses in India and analysis of cases Available in URL: https://securenow.in
4. The ICN code of ethics for nurses: https://www.inc.ch

5. SCOPE OF PRACTICE FOR MIDWIVES

The Government of India (GOI) has launched the Midwifery Initiative to improve the quality-of-service provision for strengthening reproductive, maternal, and neonatal health. This initiative will create a new cadre of "Nurse Practitioner in Midwifery" (NPM) who are skilled in accordance with International Confederation of Midwives (ICM) competencies, knowledgeable and competent in providing skilled, compassionate, respectful, women cantered care. These midwifery services will primarily be provided through 'Midwife Led Care Units' (MLCUs). One of the key components of establishing the NPM cadre and embedding them in the health system is a clear "Scope of Practice" which also guides their education, regulation, and ongoing professional development to ensure optimal midwifery care.

Definition of a Midwife (International Context)

The ICM defines a Midwife as: " a person who has successfully completed a midwifery education programme that is duly recognized in the country where it is located and that is based on the International Confederation of Midwives (ICM) Essential Competencies for basic midwifery practice and the framework of the ICM Global Standards for Midwifery Education; has acquired the requisite qualifications to be registered and/or legally licensed to practice midwifery and use the title 'midwife' and who demonstrates competency in the practice of midwifery." (ICM).

Definition of a Nurse Practitioner Midwife (NPM) (Indian Context) An NPM is one who has successfully completed the 18 months' Nurse Practitioner in Midwifery training program designed by the Indian Nursing Council (INC) based on the ICM essential competencies for basic midwifery practice and recognized in India by the Ministry of Health and Family Welfare, Government of India, and who will be registered and licensed to practice midwifery in high caseload facilities across the country under the title 'Nurse Practitioner Midwife', upon demonstrating competency in the practice of midwifery. The NPM is a responsible and accountable professional who works in partnership with women to provide the necessary support, respectful care and advice to women and their families during pregnancy, childbirth and the postpartum period

1. The NPM will function primarily in the MLCUs alongside Comprehensive Emergency Obstetric and Neonatal Care (CEmONC) centres, under the overall supervision of the Obstetrician at the facility, as envisaged by Government of India(GoI). MLCUs shall promote normality during pregnancy, labour, birth and the postpartum period, early and timely detection of complications, carry out first line emergency measures, refer and facilitate access to a full range of medical and surgical care as well as provide preventive care

2. The NPM will be able to competently perform the full scope of practice as per the education and training curriculum laid down by INC in accordance with MoHFW regulations and guidelines.

3. They are fully responsible and accountable to provide care within their defined scope of practice in the country

4. They have the authority within their area of expertise to:

■ **Educate and counsel women and their families on birth preparedness and complication readiness (BPCR), care prior to, during and after pregnancy, care of the healthy newborn, healthy timing and spacing of pregnancy including postpartum family planning and other health**

■ **Advocate for women's needs, autonomy and agency**

■ **Order and interpret diagnostic procedures and laboratory tests**

■ **Prescribe selected medications**

■ **Assess and triage women at the time of admission and refer the high-risk cases to the Obstetric Led Care Unit (OLCU)**

■ **Provide care for women, and their newborns according to best evidence during normal pregnancy, labour, birth and the postnatal period including identification and initial management of selected complications during this period**

■ **Consult with and refer to other professionals and services for care outside of their scope of practice and ensure continuity of care from preconception to the postnatal period**

■ **Document and review provision of care**

Scope of practice for midwives

The primary function of NPMs is to act professionally within their work environment to ensure the wellbeing of childbearing woman and her newborn. NPMs should instil confidence in women for their capabilities in childbirth and empower them to assume responsibility for their health, to enable them to learn for themselves, to build on their strengths and to access services in a timely way.

Scope of Practice for ME & NPM Applies to specialized midwifery care competencies gained through the 18 months educational program that is competency-based education (Annexure3). This document is combined with and adapted from key competencies for essential midwifery practice (ICM 2019) and sets out the contours for NPM practice in India as follows:

A. Pre-pregnancy Care (Sexual and Reproductive Health)

• Provide Family planning counselling and services

• Provide Pre-conception care and counselling

• Perform measures in prevention and screening for Sexually Transmitted Infections and advice treatment based on the syndromic management approach.

B. Antenatal care

• Determine health status of pregnant women

• Detect and confirm pregnancy, estimate gestational age from history, physical examination and advice on laboratory test from the recommended list of investigations

• Monitor the progression of pregnancy

• Assess foetal and maternal wellbeing

• Promote and support healthy behaviours that improve women's wellbeing including ANC exercises. • Detect, manage, and refer women with complicated pregnancies

• Provide counselling to the women and their family on the following: Preparation of birth preparedness and complication readiness plan

---

■ Antenatal education and anticipatory guidance related to pregnancy, birth, breastfeeding, parenthood, postpartum family planning and change in the family.

■ Self-care in normal pregnancy at every contact

■ Pregnancy options and care to women with unintended or mistimed pregnancy

■ Safe abortion services and post abortion care to womens

■ Post-partum & Post- aborted Family Planning Methods

C. Care during labour and birth (Intrapartum Care)

- **Confirm onset of labour**
- **Provide supportive respectful care to all women in normal labour at term and in immediate postnatal period 2(e.g., facilitate alternate birthing positions, birth companionship chosen by women, facilitate informed choices/rights-based care)**
- **Identify complications during labour, childbirth and the immediate postpartum period, and provide immediate management3 and referral when indicated**
- **Assist physiological birthing processes leading to a safe birth and active management of the third stage of labour for the prevention of postpartum hemorrhage**
- **Provide immediate essential newborn care (warmth, early initiation of breastfeeding, delayed cord clamping, Vitamin K, eye, and cord care)**
- **Perform neonatal resuscitation when indicated**
- **Identify newborn complications, perform immediate management and when indicated, initiate a timely referral**
- **Perform and repair episiotomy for evidence-based indications with the woman's consent**
- **Repair perineal, vaginal and vulval lacerations (excluding 3rd /4th degree or complicated tears)**

D. Ongoing care of women and newborns (Postpartum Care)

Provide postnatal care which focuses on continuing health assessment of women and infant, health education, intake of IFA & Calcium, support for breastfeeding, detection of complications and provision of family planning services.

Scope of practice for midwives

- Identify postpartum complications in the women and newborn, provide immediate management and when indicated, initiate referral promptly
- Counsel on postpartum family planning services
- Provide anticipatory guidance to the woman and her family on prompt recognition of danger signs in both the mother and baby and seek immediate care

Additional Roles & Responsibility for ME In addition to the above-mentioned roles illustrated from points A to D, the ME's will have the following additional responsibilities:

- Play a dual role of imparting training to the NPMs at State Midwifery Training Institutes alongside performing clinical practice themselves
- Supervise the NPMs during their clinical practice sessions
- Mentor and handhold the NPMs during and after the training

Principles of Collaborative Care

While NPMs are a specialized cadre of nurse-midwives in India and are fully responsible and accountable for care within their defined scope of practice, they work within a health care system that recognizes the need for consultation, collaboration, and referral between health care professionals. Collaboration between NPMs, Obstetricians, Paediatricians and Medical Officers In-charge (MO) requires confidence, trust and effective communication. When effective collaboration occurs, the specialists can extend their contribution to the care of women and newborns experiencing complications and requiring specialized care. NPMs can also be involved in the care of women with high-risk pregnancies, pregnancy related complications and women/newborns as a part of multidisciplinary team

REFERENCE:

1. Scope of Practice for Midwifery Educator & Nurse Practitioner Midwife, Ministry of Health & Family Welfare, Government of India, June 2021. Available in URL http://www.indiannursingcouncil.org

6. TRENDS IN MIDWIFERY

The practice of medicine and obstetrics is constantly changing as new research emerges. And the American College of Obstetricians and Gynecologists (ACOG), which is the professional organization that most obstetricians look to for guidelines in order to take the best care of the mother and the baby during pregnancy, plays a big role in setting up new trends and practices.

New Trends in Maternity's & Midwifery Nursing is rapidly changing the world, that required professionals to remain up to date in order to react to new any developments as they occur. High-quality of care, evidence-based practice is a key strategy for improving maternal and newborn health and a critical component in the continuum of care.

New teaching methods for practical training are proved to have lots of benefits in the professional training of nurses. The realistic conditions in simulation laboratories are reflecting real hospital and patient's care, communication with patient and hospital staff, discussion, and analysis of all students' activities.

The WHO sustainable development goal of 2030 (Health of Mother and Child)

1. Reduce the rate of maternal mortality.

2. Reduce the rate of fetal and infant death.

3. Reduce preterm birth.

4. Reduce cesarean births among low-risk women.

1. To Reduce the rate of maternal mortality

a. The WHO near-miss approach:

The WHO defines a maternal near- miss approach case as a women who nearly died but survived a complication that occurred during pregnancy, childbirth or within 42 days of termination of pregnancy.

Implementing The WHO Near-Miss Approach: The complete WHO near-miss approach is best implemented in three steps:

---

(1) baseline assessment (or reassessment).
(2) situation analysis; and
(3) interventions for improving health care.

Implementing the approach within a health-care facility

There are, five potentially life-threatening conditions are used as part of the inclusion criteria set: severe postpartum haemorrhage, severe pre-eclampsia, eclampsia, sepsis/severe systemic infection, and ruptured uterus. Diseases or conditions that may be relevant to a severe maternal outcome but are not part of the chain of events leading to that severe maternal outcome should be specified under contributory/associated conditions.

Critical interventions are those that are required in the management of life-threatening and potentially life-threatening conditions. In this guide, blood transfusion, interventional radiology, and laparotomy (including hysterectomy and other emergency surgical interventions in the abdominal cavity but excluding caesarean section) fall into this category.

Admission to intensive care unit is defined as admission to a unit that provides 24-hour medical supervision and can provide mechanical ventilation and continuous vasoactive drug support.

Maternal death is defined as death of a woman while pregnant or within 42 days of termination of pregnancy, irrespective of the duration and the site of the pregnancy, from any cause related to or aggravated by the pregnancy or its management, but not from accidental or incidental causes.

Maternal near-miss case is defined as "a woman who nearly died but survived a complication that occurred during pregnancy, childbirth or within 42 days of termination of pregnancy". In practical terms, women are considered near miss cases when they survive life-threatening conditions (i.e., organ dysfunction).

Severe maternal outcomes are maternal near miss cases and maternal deaths.

Process indicators are those that assess the processes of health care. In this guide, process indicators are those that assess the use of key interventions for the prevention and management of severe complications. Data on the use of key interventions provide information on the implementation status of evidence-based recommendations.

Sentinel units are structures in the facility that are likely to provide care to women with severe complications related to pregnancy, childbirth or postpartum (e.g., maternal high-risk wards, high-dependency or intensive care units, surgical recovery room, emergency or facility-arrival room, blood bank, postabortion care units, and others).

b. Maternal waiting home:

Many women in low- and middle-income countries face the challenges of inaccessibility of obstetric care in rural and urban areas. To minimize these problems, developing countries including India used MHW (Maternity waiting homes) as an alternative to increase accessibility of obstetric care services.

MHW are homes built in the compound or near to health centres that provides standard medical and emergency obstetric care services.

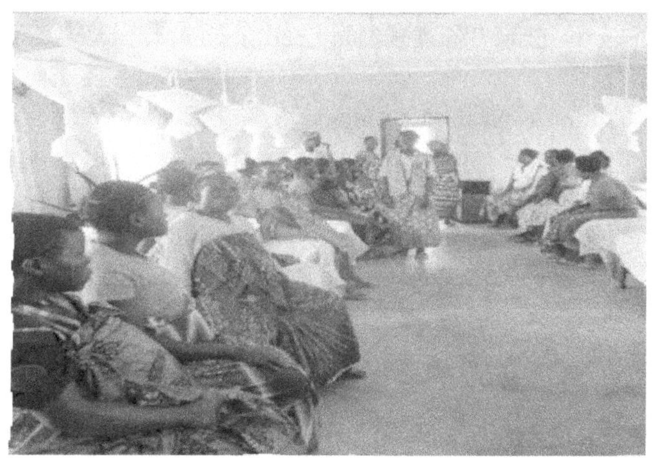

Figure 16: Maternity Waiting home

c. **Post-partum butterfly:**

It is simple cost-effective device developed by Professor Andrew Weeks as a treatment method for postpartum haemorrhage. Postpartum Haemorrhage (PPH) is a significant cause of maternal morbidity and mortality. The most common cause is the inability of the uterus to contract adequately after childbirth. So, the obstetricians attempt for the bimanual Compression (BMC), one hand is placed within the vagina and the other hand is on abdominal wall to compress the uterus. It is effective, but it is effective, but very uncomfortable for the woman. This PPH Butterfly device that replicate BMC without inserting a hand vaginally, it also helps in diagnosing the source of bleeding.

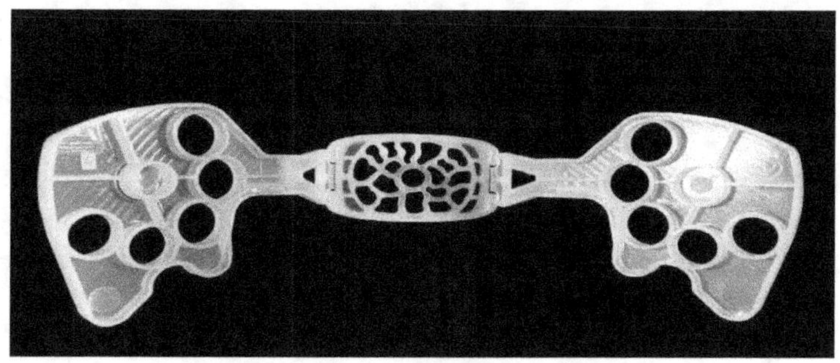

Figure 17: PPH Butterfly

d. Transvaginal Bakri Balloon replacement:

The Bakri balloon is an intrauterine device indicated to reduce or control PPH temporarily when conservative treatment is warranted. It appears to be an effective alternative for the management of acute PPH refractory to medical treatment and requires minimal training to use. The device consists of a silicone balloon connected to a catheter of the same material. The collapsed balloon is inserted into the uterine cavity, and when it is inflated with liquid it conforms to the shape of the cavity and stops the bleeding. The blood drains through the central lumen of the catheter, and blood loss can then be evaluated. The main advantages described for the Bakri balloon are its easy transvaginal or transabdominal insertion, which can bring about rapid tamponade of the uterine cavity, simplify control of the bleeding and avoid the need for other more invasive procedures, such as hysterectomy

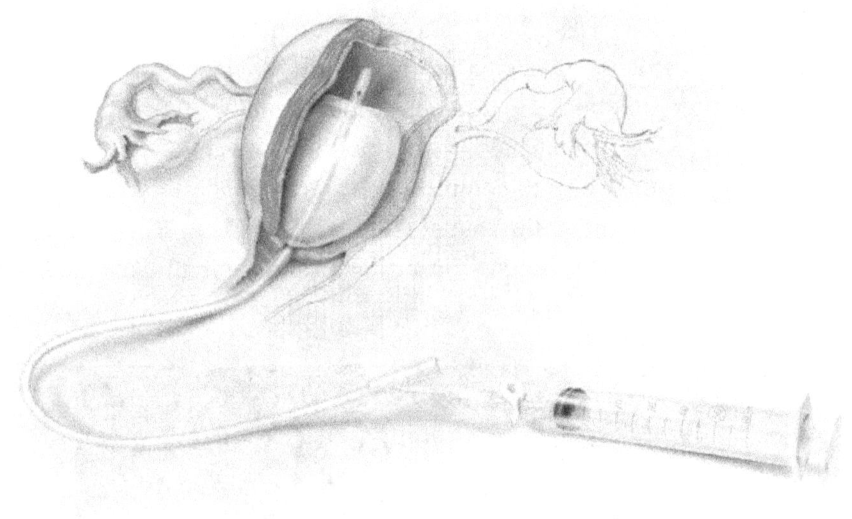

Figure 18: Transvaginal Bakri Balloon replacement

e. LUCAS External Cardiac Compressor:

The LUCAS (Lund University Cardiopulmonary Assisted System) CPR device is a mobile tool for conducting chest compressions. Traditionally CPR was conducted by a health care professional. However, in recent times, there has been a mechanical compression device that perform CPR. Compression is carried out by an automated machine that is powered electrically or utilizes air pressure. Statistics indicate that the tool administer CPR first aid, can even perform better than a person.

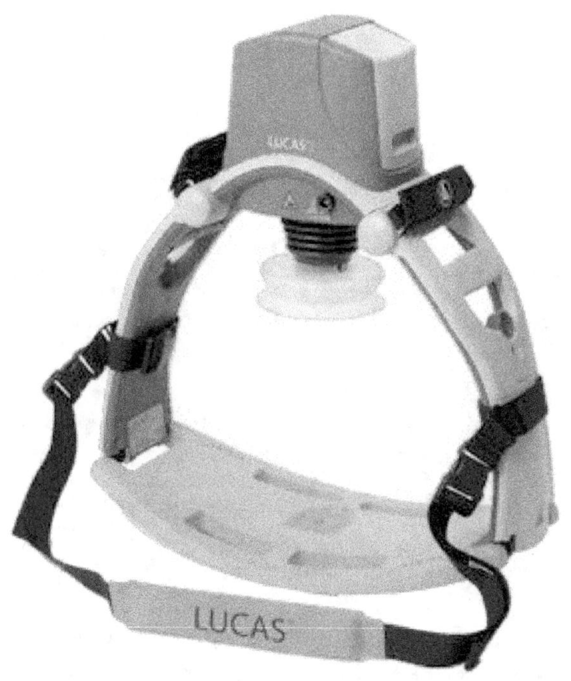

Figure 19: LUCAS External Cardiac Compressor

2. To Reduce the rate of fetal and infant death:

a) Wireless fetal monitoring.

The Monica Novi™ Wireless Patch System uses Bluetooth technology to record the baby's heartbeat, the mom's heartbeat, and the frequency and duration of contractions. Novi is applied to a mother's belly with a stick-on patch, with no wires or belts.

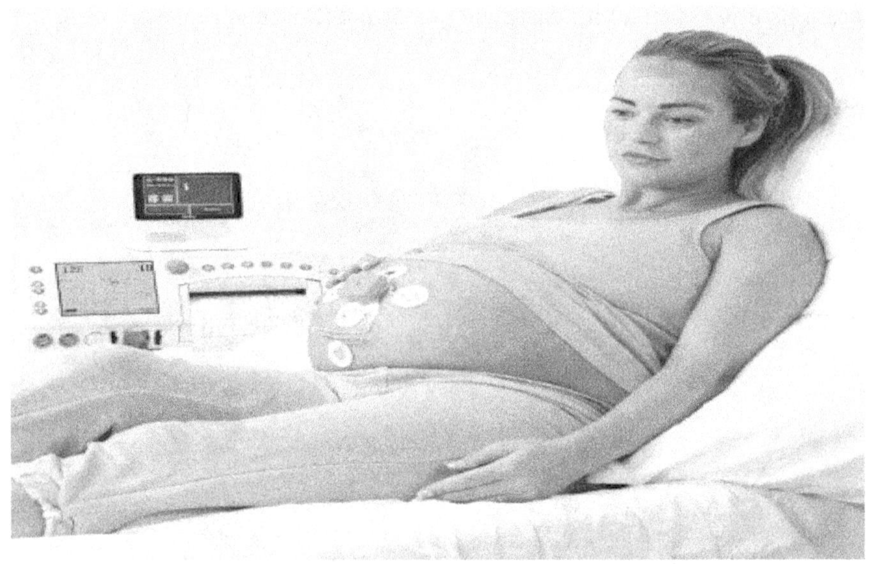

Figure 20: Wireless foetal monitoring

b. Foetal Monitoring using smartphone

In this method, a smart phone using a cheap portable doppler ultrasound connected to the phone. The mother can use the system to monitor FHR and foetal activity. Once the monitoring is completed, the FHR and the corresponding activity indicators can be transferred to a medical team in a hospital or health centre is able to make a decision quickly as to further examinations of the foetus and the pregnant mother are required.

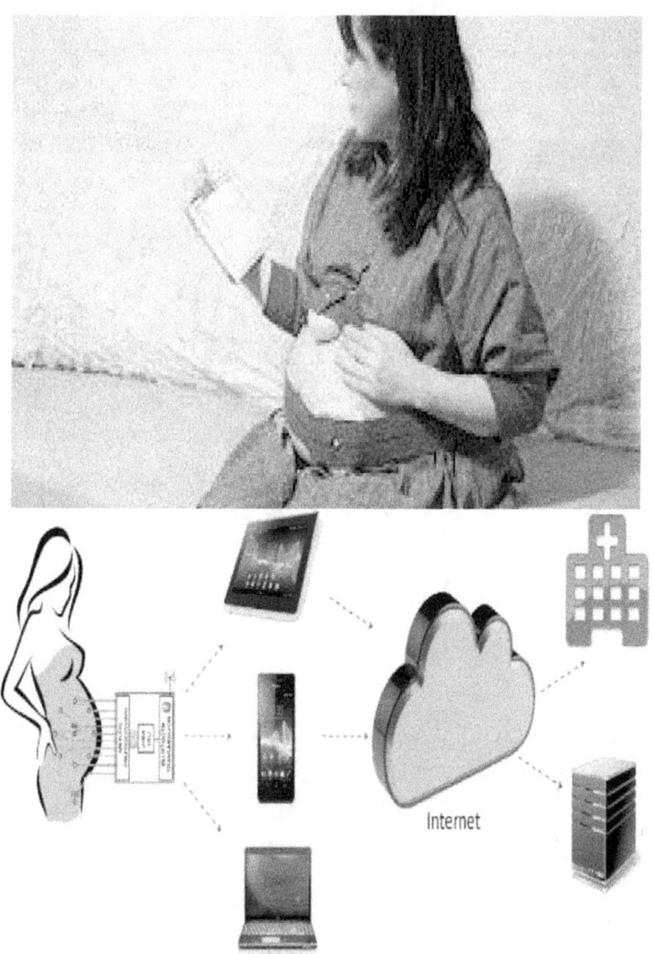

Figure 21 & 22: Foetal monitoring using smartphone & process of transformation

C. Non-invasive prenatal testing (Cell-free DNA screening).

Screening for foetal chromosol abnormalities during pregnancy is an essential part of obstetrical care. NIPT (Non-invasive prenatal testing) is a safe screening test which can be offered to all pregnant woman and that is more accurate than the blood based and USG based test to identify fetus with trisomy.

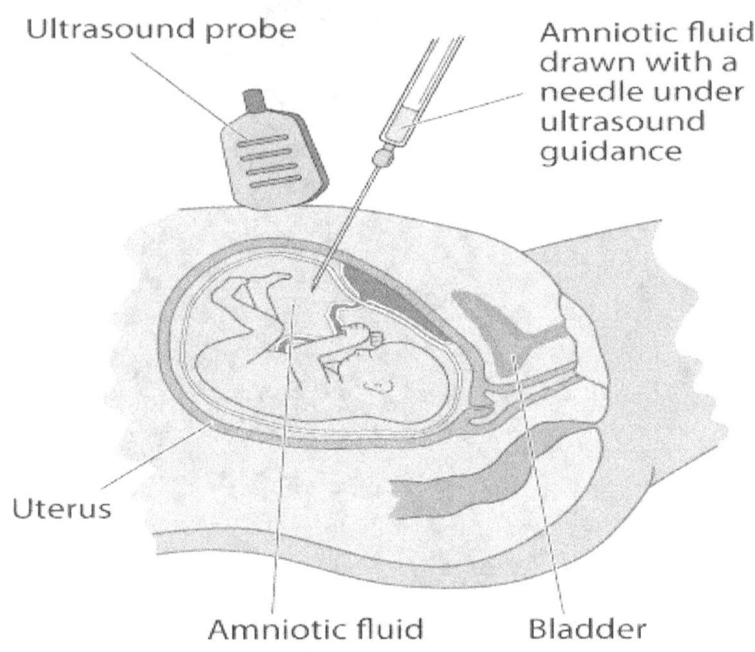

Figure 23: Non-Invasive Prenatal Testing (NIPT)

d.   Vaginal seeding.

Vaginal seeding is the practice of wiping a baby's mouth, face and skin with its mother's vaginal fluids after C-section. This process transfers vaginal microbes to the baby to help establish the baby's own microbiome to promote good health and fight disease. But the practice has some risks, and healthcare providers don't recommend it due to some risks associated with this procedure.

3. To Reduce preterm births

a)   WHO approach to reduce preterm

b)   Maternal progesterone supplementation.

c)   Cervical Encirclage for incompetent cervix

d) Treatment of intra-uterine infection.

e) Prevent exposure to cigarette smoking.

f) Improvement of maternal nutrition.

g) Lifestyle modification to ameliorate maternal stress.

h) (Omega-3 fatty acid)

4. Reduce cesarean births among low-risk women

---

a. **Second opinion have to obtained for performing caesarean except emergency LSCS.**
b. **Changing the local culture and attitudes of doctors regarding the interventions to reduce CSR (Caesarean section rates) across indications, across community, and academic settings.**
c. **Women with uncomplicated pregnancy should be offered induction of labour beyond 41 weeks which will reduce perinatal mortality and likelihood of CS.**
d. **Foetal malpresentation should be assessed and documented to allow for external cephalic version to be offered.**
e. **VABC should be offered and encouraged for all patients unless there is a separate complicated factor that justifies CS.**
f. **Public awareness should be created about risk and benefits of CS, as compared with Vaginal birth.**

New technology in maternity & newborn health nursing:

a. Robotic Gynecological Surgery

- **Robotics is a new field in surgery especially in complex operations are involved in taking a patient's vitals, medical history and updating medical records**
- **The robotic nurse plays an essential role in a successful robotic surgery. As part of the robotic surgical team, each one of the robotic nursing team "nurse coordinator, scrub-nurse and circulating-nurse" has a certain job description to ensure maximum patient's safety and robotic surgical efficiency.**
- **Well-structured training programs should be offered to the robotic nurse to be well prepared, feel confident, and maintain high-quality of care. Uses in, Hysterectomy & tubal ligations., Removal of fibroid tumors & Myomectomy, Removal of ovarian cysts & ovarian tumors. Infertility surgery, Endometriosis surgery, Genital Prolapse surgery.**

---

b. The Vita Heat During Labor

- The Vita HEAT is a portable system that moves with the woman throughout entire labour process.
- Portable, under-body system delivers warmth and helps improve women satisfaction &comfort. Also, use as non-pharmacology pain relievers.

c. Virtual Reality (VR) Eases Labor Pains

Virtual reality (VR) is one of the newest non-pharmacological labor pain managements is a new technology can help parturient learns pain management skills like breathing exercises, meditation and visualization using VR to distract from pain perception.

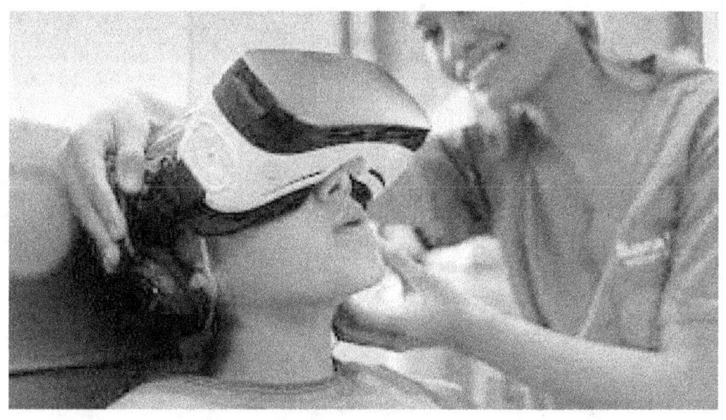

Figure 24: Virtual Reality (VR)

d.　**Lactation Massaging Bra (The Lilu):**

It is used to stimulate milk glands and help to achieve let down by using wireless, researchable remote. The Lilu is a powered bra which has massager. It is used to relieve milk from blocked lactiferous ducts. So, the Lilu is efficiently used for Breast engorgement.

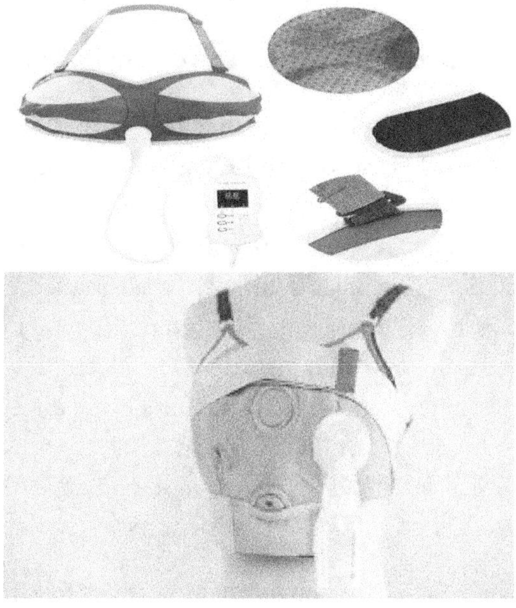

Figure 25 &26 Lactation massaging Bra(Lila) with mill collection bottle

e. Clearblue Digital Pregnancy Test

Clearblue Digital Pregnancy Test is a highly effective and advanced digital pregnancy test. It is more than 99% accurate at detecting fertility. **Clearblue** is the first one-step home ovulation test, enabling women to measure their surge in LuteinizingHormone (LH) to determine their most fertile days.

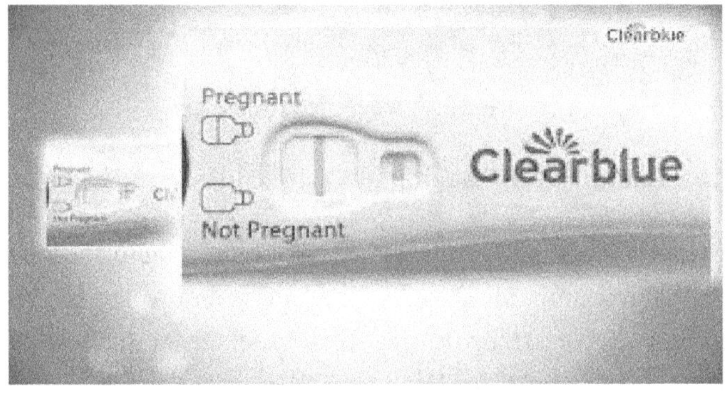

Figure 27: Digital pregnancy test kit

f. Transcutaneous Electric Nerve Stimulation:

Transcutaneous electrical nerve stimulation (TENS) is a method of pain relief involving the use of mild electrical current. It can be used during labour process to reduce pain and also in postnatal period to prevent postnatal complications. A TENS machine is a small, battery-operated device which has leads connected to sticky pads called electrodes. The electrical impulses block the pain signals going to spinal cord and brain which may reduce pain and relax muscles. The electrodes can be applied to the area where it presents. During labour, one pair of electrodes is applied at either side of the spinal (C_{12}-T_{11}). Later stages of labour one pair of electrodes is applied at (S_2-S_3) another pair of electrode over symphysis pubis. This gives local analgesic effect.

Kegel exerciser and muscle stimulator for women to strengthen pelvic floor. It is new pelvic floor muscle trainer to help women with post-partum complications and incontinence

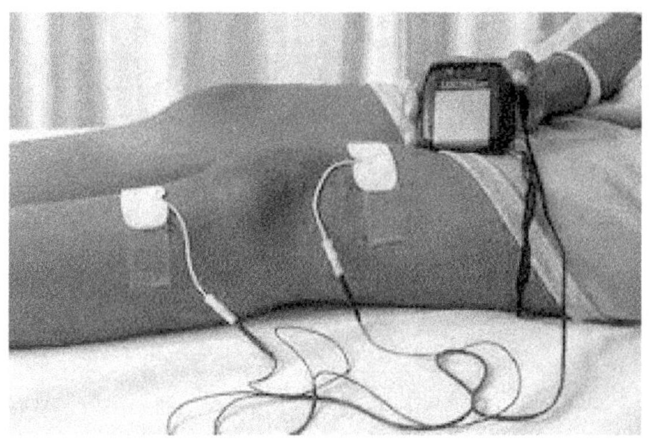

Figure 28: Transcutaneous Electric Nerve Stimulation (TENS)

Benefits:

- Pelvic floor trainers: helps women prevent bladder leaks, urges to urinate, urinary incontinence,and other pelvic floor issues.

- Better bladder control: Regain and maintain bladder control women of all ages and sizes can avoid bladder leaks. And this

- Easy-to-use muscle toners: It is stimulator technology will do the pelvic exercises automatic. Apply lubricant onto the stimulator and place device comfortably inside the vagina, with the silver parts facing toward their hips. Only 20 minutes a day can help women get results effortlessly and proven results.

A Contraceptive Computer Chip (Remote Control)

- A contraceptive computer chip that can be controlled by remote control has been developed. The chip is implanted under a woman's skin, releasing a small dose of levonorgestrel daily. Safe, effective, long-term birth control.A small electric charge melts an ultra-thin seal around the levonorgestrel, releasing the 30 mcg dose into the body for and this will happen every day for 16 years, but can be stopped at any times by using a wireless remote control. The device measures 20 x 20 x 7 millimeters, and it is designed to be implanted under the skin of the buttocks, upper arm, or abdomen.

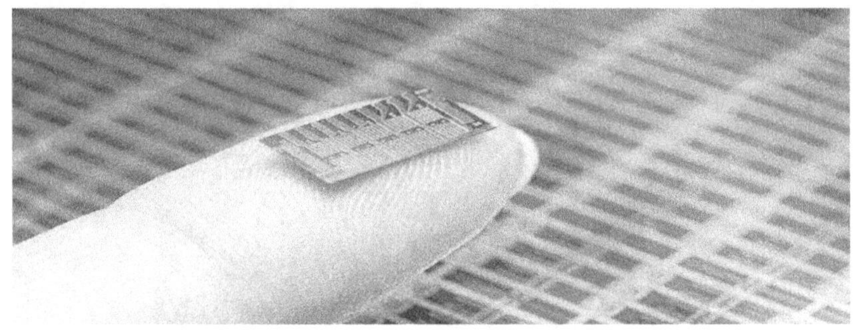

Figure 29: Contraceptive chip

Other trends in obstetrics and gynaecology

Currents trends in obstetrical nursing are follows as technological advances increased cost of high- tech care, changing patterns of childbirth, prenatal risk factors, and family centred care, rising caesarean birth rates early discharge and role of fathers in childbirth.

a. Delayed Umbilical Cord Clamping After Birth

Delayed cord clamping means waiting anywhere from 30 seconds to a few minutes to clamp and cut the umbilical cord instead of immediately following delivery. By delaying cord clamping, baby will get additional blood from mom, which contains oxygen-carrying iron stores. ACOG has recently (2017) recommended that in healthy infants, cord clamping should be delayed at least 30-60 seconds.

b. Jet Hydrotherapy/ Laboring in Water

The women's body is immersed in tank of water, with help of mechanical device air is injected to produce bubbles which stimulates nipples of the women to produce endorphin. Endorphin gives natural analgesic effect. Immersion in water can help decrease the need for an epidural or other pain medication in women with healthy, uncomplicated pregnancies. However, once it's time to begin pushing it's best to get out of the tub because delivering baby in the water hasn't been well studied and there have been reports of serious complications.

c. Cell-Free DNA Genetic Screening

Cell-free DNA screening is the newest way to screen for genetic problems in the baby. This is a simple blood test that can detect pieces of the baby's DNA in mom's blood to determine if there may be a problem with the pregnancy.

d. Immediate Postpartum IUD Insertion

An IUD is one of the most reliable methods of birth control available. However now, immediately following birth, an IUD can be inserted, eliminating the need for an extra visit and an extra procedure.

e. Limiting Interventions During Low-Risk Labor

Physicians have gotten a bad reputation for unnecessary interventions during labor and delivery. While there are times that interventions are needed for a safe delivery, limiting unnecessary interventions can also be beneficial. They are encouraging the use of doulas, changing positions during labor, intermittent monitoring, and non-pharmacologic methods of pain control in conjunction with women's birth plans.

f. Terminology

An ACOG Committee Opinion issued in December 2005 expressed concern about on-going use of the terms "foetal distress" and "birth asphyxia," recommending abolition of the term "birth asphyxia" as a nonspecific diagnosis and replacing "foetal distress" with the term "non-reassuring foetal status."

g. APGAR Scores: Not Predictive

Apgar scores have been used since the 1950s to describe the condition of neonates. ACOG advocates that its use be restricted to the labour & delivery room and not beyond as an indication or report of an acute intra-partum hypoxic event. Low Apgar scores at one and five minutes neither indicate hypoxia nor predict long-term neurologic outcomes.

h.   Limitations Of Electronic Foetal Monitoring

EFM has its limitations. An ACOG Practice Bulletin issued in December 2005 reviewed some ofthese limitations:

- The false positive rate of EFM for predicting adverse outcomes is high.

The use of EFM is associated with an increase in the rate of operative deliveries (vacuum, forceps,and caesarean section. The use of EFM does not result in a reduction of cerebral palsy case rates. This same bulletin set forth the guidelines for the frequency of reviewing EFM tracings and their retention as part of the medicalrecord.

i.   The 30-Minute Interval Guideline

In 1989, ACOG's Committee on Professional Standards first established "that hospitals with obstetric   services should have the capability to begin a caesarean delivery within   30 minutes of the time that the decision is made to perform the procedure." Bloom et al   studied maternal and infant outcomes and found that a caesarean delivery with these 30 minutes interval guideline does not prevent all poor infant outcomes ad "by no means guarantees infant safety."

J. Effective Anesthesia for Obstetric Patients:

The introduction of combined spinal– epidural anesthesia (CSEA) offers benefits of
both techniques. CSEA also offers the prospect of reducing the anesthetic failure rate of either technique used alone.

k. Stem Cell Therapy and Cord Blood Banking:

Stem Cell technology has taken the world by storm. The potential benefits are innumerable and newer uses are coming on over the horizon. It has already shown promise in treating over 75 diseases like the following:

- **Cardiac repair**
- **Treatment of type II Diabetes Mellitus**
- **Treatment of neurological injury like- brain injury, Alzheimer's Disease,**
- **Huntington's Disease,Amyotrophic Lateral Sclerosis, to name a few.**
- **Malignancies**
- **Regenerative medicine- of the joint, tissue, or organ**
- **Gene Therapy.**
- **Patient awareness campaigns are underway and baby's cord blood is need to**
- **harvest these stem cells a relatively easy means of cell procurement. Stem cell therapy will be a cornucopia of benefits to humanity, virtually unlimited in its future potential. That future begins now.**

High Risk Obstetrics- The Future:

Investments in obstetric patient safety maximize their return by preventing high-severity claims. Somepatient safety approaches that hold promise include:

- **Obstetrics Rapid Response Teams**
- **Medical emergency preparedness strategies, such as training, stocking appropriate supplies, early warning systems, and specialized first responders.**
- **Team training using crew resource management techniques borrowed from the military and the airline industry**
- **Commercially available clinical informatics systems that promote patient safety at the patient's bedside and in real time**

- **Health care professionals to determine which format (send staff to a simulation center, develop in- house simulation program, and develop a consortium of hospitals that run a simulation program, or use a mobile simulation program) is best for them.**

GYNAECOLOGY:

Gynecological disease directly affects the quality of life of women in different ways and
in varying degrees, highlighting the value and importance of patient assessed health status measures to evaluate the subjective severity and treatment efficacy of common gynecological conditions.

Treatment Of Menorrhagia:

The Nova sure System is the latest generation of devices that treat the entire inside of the uterus (endometrial cavity) at once. The procedure does not require any incisions and does not require hospitalization. A slender device is inserted through the cervix under local anesthesia with sedation, or general anesthesia. Once it is in place, treatment time averages 90 seconds. Most women can resume most of their normal activities in a day or two. A major advantage of Nova sure is that hormonal pre- treatment is not needed, and it can be done at any time of the cycle.

Treatment Of Fibroids:

Bilateral embolization of uterine arteries

The latest in the treatment of large symptomatic fibroids is embolization of the uterine arteries, but it is being done in only some centers as it is still in the evaluation phase. It has been shown that embolization of the uterine arteries with polyvinyl alcohol particles introduced transfemorally by catheter can significantly reduce the size of large fibroids (60%-65%) and produce significant symptomatic improvement or complete resolution of symptoms.

1. Robotic Myomectomy

This is an upcoming trend in the surgical management of fibroids of the uterus. An example of onesuch is the one done with the Da Vinci Surgical Robot.

2. Hormone Replacement Therapy (HRT)

HRT that can be sprayed into the nose could be the answer for women who have trouble with traditional forms of treatment. The estrogen nasal spray has been hailed the biggest breakthrough since hormonal replacement therapy patches were invented 20 years ago.

3. In Contraception

Minor procedure units for gynecology, with one stop investigation and treatment (including ultrasonography and hysteroscopy), and early pregnancy assessment units, where bleeding in early pregnancy can be dealt with rapidly and sympathetically, are becoming more commonplace. The prolonged life expectancy of menopausal women and their higher expectations for health have encouraged new developments in hormone replacement therapy.

New trends in education of maternal and newborn health nursing

Implementation of the new practical teaching methods, simulation of the methods such as the Group strategy (Jigsaw strategy), Practical workshop, interact evaluation, Group discussion, Mind mapping, Case studies, Problem/concept mapping, Role play, E-learning, and Problem-based learning in practical training could help improve quality of the educational process in midwifery.

1. Telecommunication

Nurses, who deliver, manage, and coordinate care and services using telecommunication technology are determined to be providing telenursing. Tele-nursing may occur via interactive video discussions enabling visualization of the person to determine the appropriate care or education required.

Telecommunication for day-to-day during high-risk pregnancy tests and steps, including:

- Electronic medical record (EMR) consultations: Reviewing and making recommendations for carebased on a patient's medical history and test results, all of which are detailed in the EMR.
- Genetic counseling: Talking with patients about their risk factors for passing genetic conditions to theirbabies.
- Videoconferencing: The doctor and patient can discuss findings during ultrasound examinations face-to-face over video.
- Virtual rounding: Being at an inpatient's bedside across the state through mobile device technology.

Modern and effective teaching methods in midwifery education, which are done in accordance with proclaimed goals of study program in midwifery, profile of graduate, profile of midwife and final midwives' competencies are necessary for final reform and for creation of professional with full of appropriate knowledge and skills.

2. Practical Workshop

The practical workshop is a form of educational activity in which the lecturer/assistant prepares topics, objectives, content, steps of the educational process and a variety of techniques (brainstorming, feedback) for students to use their own knowledge and experience to acquire skills that will use in practice. The goal of practical workshop is to train and strengthen already acquired knowledge and skills.

3. Case Studies

Case study is a description of emergency/interesting clinical case/ disease. It is used as a form of presentation, particularly in some biomedical and social sciences. Case studies have potential for measuring application of knowledge, analysis, problem-solving and evaluative skills. This method allows students to apply theory to practical situations.

4. Training With Simulator Mannequins in The Laboratories

Learning with simulator mannequins in nursing is the combination of interactive simulations of real- life clinical scenarios for the purpose of nursing training, education and assessment.

5. Nursing Process

The aim of this method is to evaluate the patient's medical condition, actual and potential health problems, the level of health care, make a plan to assess the patient's needs and provide specific nursing interventions to meet those needs. This process consists of the following phases: assessing the health problems of the patient, diagnosis, intervention planning, implementation and evaluation of interventions provided by nursing care.

6. Mind Mapping

Mind mapping joins the critical thinking, case-based learning, and press students to make a visual scheme how to solve the patient's problem. Concept maps include concepts, usually enclosed in circles or boxes of some type and relationships between concepts or propositions, indicated by a connecting lineand linking words between concepts.

7. Problem-Based Learning

Principles of problem-based learning (PBL) are based on the fact that students are actively participating in planning, organizing and evaluating the problem-solving process. Objectives of theproblem-based learning process are knowledge (theoretical and clinical), skills (scientific reasoning, critical appraisal, information literacy, self-directed lifelong learning) and attitudes (value of teamwork, interpersonal skills, importance of psycho-social skills.

8. Mind Mapping

Mind mapping joins the critical thinking, case-based learning and press students to make a visual scheme how to solve the patient's problem. Concept maps include concepts, usually enclosed in circles or boxes of some type and relationships between concepts or propositions, indicated by a connecting lineand linking words between concepts.

9. Problem-Based Learning

Principles of problem-based learning (PBL) are based on the fact that students are actively participating in planning, organizing and evaluating the problem solving process. Objectives of theproblem-based learning process are knowledge (theoretical and clinical), skills (scientific reasoning, critical appraisal, information literacy, self-directed lifelong learning) and attitudes (value of teamwork, interpersonal skills, importance of psycho-social issues.

Medical Science is a dynamic cornucopia of latest and more innovative developments and improvements of current techniques and therapies. With better patient awareness and an environment of unrelenting litigation we have found ourselves strenuously trying to balance sound judgement on the part of the physician and well-informed consent for related treatment plans for the patient. So, the final word lies in the fact that ultimately the most effective way to improve healthcare is to make it more collaborative. It is important for maternity nurses to recognize that new technology help to improve maternal and new-born health. Building skills, continuous training is very important to improve maternal health and improve quality of care.

REFERENCE

1. Reeder, Martin, Koniak-Griffin Maternity Nursing, Family, Newborn and Women's Healthcare, Editor-A V Raman, 19th Edition (2014), Published by Wolters Kluwer (India)Pvt. Ltd., New Delhi, Page no: 2- 12

2. Bobak Jenson, Maternity & Gynecologic Care, Mosby, 5th edition-1992, page: 7-10

3. Dickson Silverman, Maternity-infant care, Mosby, 2nd Edition-1993, page: 7-10

4. Erna E. Ziezel, Obstetric Nursing, Newyork Mac- Millan, 8th edition-1992, page: 53- 57

5. Lynna Y. Littleton-Gibbs et al, Maternity Nursing Care, 2nd Edition-2013, page: 12,13

6. Emily Slone Mc Kinney et al, Maternal-Child Nursing, W. B. Saunders Company, page: 6-

7. F. Gary Cunningham et al, Williams Obstetrics, 22nd Edition, 2005, page: 9-12

8. Susan L. Ward et al, Maternal-Child Nursing Care, F. A. Davis Company, 2009, page:11-16

9. Tabassum parvez, Journal of International Medical Sciences Academy (JIMSA), July-September 2012 vol. 25 no. 3, page no: 155-157

10. Stefania Andrascikova et al. Journal of Clinical Obstetrics, Gynecology & Infertility,2017, vol. 1, issues. 1, page no: 1-3

11. https://www.mother.ly/lifestyle/5-obstetrics-trends-

12. 4.Lilu massage bra Available in URL https: www.wearlilu.com

13. 5.How to reduce CS rate Available in URL http://www.slideshare.net

14. 6.TENS. Available in URL http://www.nhs.uk.conditions

15. 7.NIPT.Available in URL http://sapac.illumina.com

16. 8.The WHO Near miss approach. Available in URL http://whqlibdoc.who.int

7. EVIDENCE BASED PRACTICE IN NURSING & MIDWIFERY

Nurses and midwives play an important role in tackling the public health challenges present in health systems across the WHO European Region. These groups of healthcare professionals collectively form the largest component of the health workforce, and are key actors in delivering effective, efficient, accessible, acceptable, patient-centred, equitable and safe health-care services. Quality health-care services require that clinical decision-making in nursing and midwifery and care coordination are based on evidence. The best available evidence should be utilized when improving aspects of quality in health care and enhancing evidence-based practice (EBP). The nursing and midwifery professions remain central to the achievement of EBP in health-care settings, particularly in standardizing and aligning health-care practices with evidence at the point of care.

Nurses and midwives should understand the meaning of EBP and facilitating factors for successful implementation. They should acknowledge the rationale for implementing EBP and strive to develop the skills to engage with evidence and apply it to daily nursing and midwifery practice.

Evidence-based health care and practice

Evidence-based health care EBHC is an umbrella concept of EBP that includes nursing, midwifery, medicine and allied health professions. It can be conceptualized as clinical decision-making that considers the feasibility, appropriateness, meaningfulness and effectiveness of healthcare practices. This may be informed by the best available evidence, the context in which care is delivered, the individual patient, and the professional judgement and expertise of the health professional. To facilitate evidence-based decision-making, all professions in health care

are to be given the opportunity to be involved in developing EBP and embedding evidence into professional practice and education . The Joanna Briggs Institute (JBI), an international nursing research organization, has developed the JBI model of EBHC. This conceptualizes: the steps of the process to achieve an evidence-based approach to clinical decision-making; how the component parts of the model are operationalized; and how they might be implemented in practice. EBHC is not a clean, linear process; at times, the process can be bi-directional, which is represented.

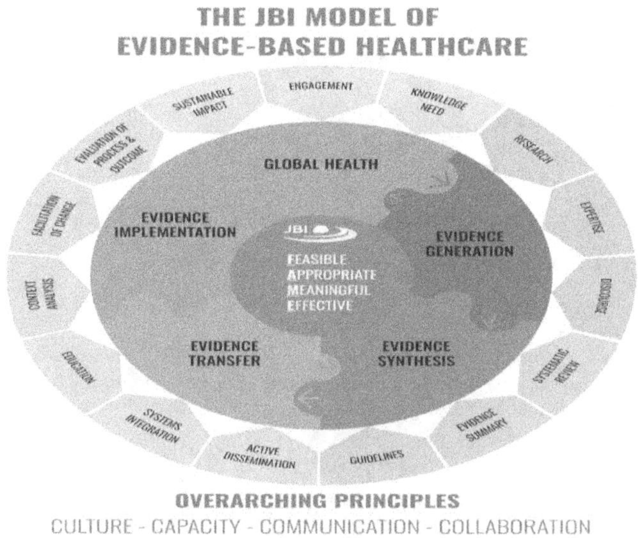

Figure 30: JBI Model for Evidence Based Practice

The central component of the model is the so-called Pebble of Knowledge, with the core phases defined as **evidence generation, evidence synthesis, evidence transfer and evidence implementation** . The feasibility, appropriateness, meaningfulness and effectiveness of various treatment options or health-care practices are to be considered in evidence-based decision-making. Global health is the ultimate goal and end point of the components of the model, which includes striving for a sustainable impact in changes to health-care practices, increased engagement and close multisectoral collaboration, and assessment of local communities' knowledgerequirements.

The core phases of the JBI model of EBHC are defined as evidence generation, evidence synthesis, evidence transfer and evidence utilization. Evidence generation includes discourse, professional expertise, and research. Research evidence is generated through original studies (primary research) and systematic reviews (secondary research). In this phase, systematic reviews might identify important gaps in research evidence. The gold standard of evidence is recognized by many as being the randomized controlled trial, but other types have become increasingly significant in informing nursing and midwifery practice.

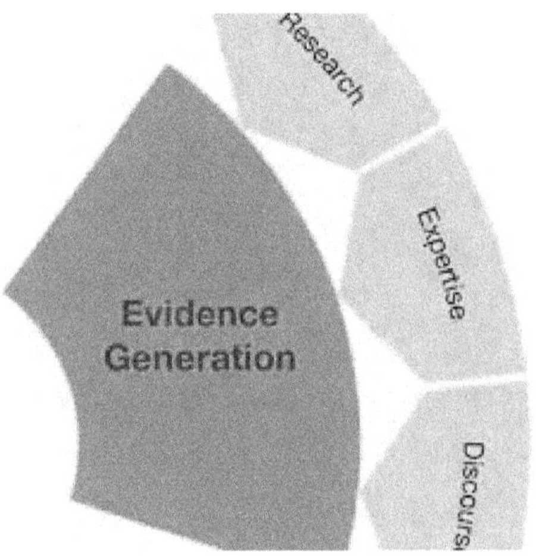

Figure 31:   Phase I- Evidence Generation

Research evidence does not always exist nurses and midwives must make decisions in care situations based on the best evidence available at any particular time. It is therefore fundamental to recognize what specific evidence is required to answer a clinical question and identify which type of evidence is available (research, experience or discourse) during the synthesis of generated evidence.

Current available evidence needs to be synthesized. Evidence synthesis is defined as: "the evaluation or analysis of research evidence and opinion on a specific topic to aid in decision making in healthcare"

Example 1. Cochrane Special Collection of Systematic Reviews The special collection brings together high-quality systematic reviews on breastfeeding to support the implementation of evidence into policy and practice. The purpose of the collection is to promote effective breastfeeding for mothers and babies through the collection of the best available evidence for use by decision-makers, health professionals, advocacy groups, and women and families.

Example 2. WHO guidelines to improve quality of antenatal care This WHO guideline includes comprehensive recommendations to reduce the risk of stillbirths and pregnancy complications and aims to give women a positive pregnancy experience. It includes recommendations for health-system interventions to improve the quality of antenatal care. The implementation of guideline recommendations can save lives, as antenatal care offers the potential to make a positive contribution to health promotion, screening and diagnosis, and disease prevention. The recommendations, which include evidence on harms and benefits, values, resources, equity, acceptability, and feasibility, are based on different sources of evidence, such as effectiveness reviews, qualitative evidence syntheses, test-accuracy reviews and mixed-method reviews, that have been assessed and synthesized.

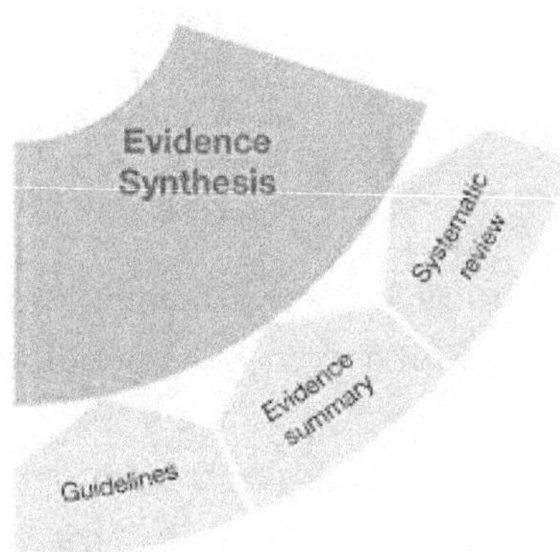

Figure32: Phase II- Evidence Synthesis

Synthesized evidence must be transferred and shared to be implemented in practice, "transfer" as meaning "a coactive, participatory process to advance access to and uptake of evidence in local contexts". Transfer enables uptake of evidence and so enables, facilitates and supports evidence implementation. Essential components of evidence transfer include active dissemination, systems integration, and education. The JBI model highlights the importance of dissemination of evidence using active methods and human communication to spread information in a format that encourages utilization. Education programmes, include continuing professional development or broader programmes, are recognized as an effective means of evidence transfer. Embedding evidence into the system, policies and procedures is necessary for decisions at all levels of organizations to be guided by evidence.

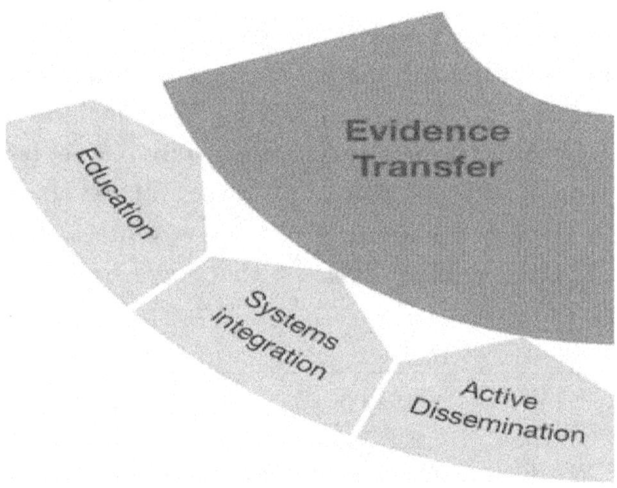

Figure 33:   Phase III- Evidence Transfer

Evidence implementation in the context of the JBI model is defined by Jordan et al. as: "a purposeful and enabling set of activities designed to engage key stakeholders with research evidence to inform decision-making and generate sustained improvement in the quality of healthcare delivery". The three main components of this phase are context analysis, facilitation of practice change, and evaluation of the process and outcome

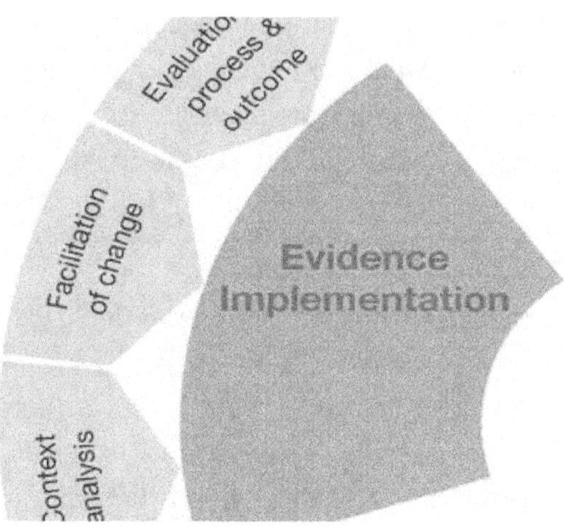

Figure 34:   Phase IV- Evidence Implementation

Prior to the adoption of an evidence-based intervention, it is necessary to design a comprehensive implementation plan that takes into consideration the principles of organizational culture, capacity, communication, and collaboration. It is vitally important to have a plan on how to monitor and evaluate, and to sustain changes made to health-care practice. Health-care professionals, educators, researchers, leaders, and policymakers have specific roles and responsibilities in the phases of implementing EBP.

Example 3. Improving patient safety through evidence-based hand-hygiene practices good hand hygiene improves patient safety and outcomes through reducing care-associated infections. The model for hand-hygiene practice evaluation and development provides evidence-based structure and guidance for systematic and consistent monitoring of hand-hygiene practices. Combining measurement of fidelity to guidelines with compliance rates reveals inconsistencies between optimal and actual hand-hygiene behaviour. Korhonen et al. evaluated hand-hygiene practices in a Finnish university hospital. Their observations suggested the compliance rate was as high as 78%, meaning that health professionals routinely used hand sanitizers.

Fidelity measures, however, showed that hand-rubbing practices were followed according to the recommendation (which states that the overall duration of hand-rubbing should last 30 seconds or more) in only 10% of cases. It is therefore necessary to measure fidelity to guidelines to gather more specific data about the implementation of EBP.

Evidence-based practice EBP is a generic term that originally arose from the field of medicine. It is universally defined as: "the conscientious, explicit and judicious use of current best evidence in making decisions about the care of the individual patient". EBP is an interdisciplinary approach to decision-making in clinical practice that includes the best available evidence, the care context, client values and preferences, and the professional judgement of the health professional. It is important for nurses and midwives to recognize that a variety of external and clinical information is needed in evidence-based clinical decision-making. Further, clinical decision-making is affected by societal values and explicit and implicit values in the health system.

The four aspects of evidence-based decision-making process are:

- integration of the best available evidence generated by quality research.
- clinical evidence and expertise.
- patient values and preferences; and
- relevant contextual knowledge, which includes available resources and acknowledges potential resource barriers and enablers within the context of care.

The EBP movement began with the identification of the research-to-practice gap and developed into a movement in which the principles of EBP have been applied to decision-making at different levels of the health system and to other fields of professional practice in health and social care, such as dentistry, nursing, midwifery, psychology, public health, radiology, social work, and policy and management. Today, EBP is considered a key component of modern health care.

The aim of evidence-based approaches to clinical practice is to deliver appropriate care in an efficient manner to the patient. EBP has been described as doing the right things right and doing things efficiently to the best standard possible, while ensuring that what is done is of known effectiveness. EBP results in quality patient outcomes when delivered in a context of caring supported by an organizational culture that supports EBP.

Currently, the concept of evidence-informed practice (EIP) is often used interchangeably with EBP without consideration of the differences or similarities. It has been argued that the evidence-based approach is too restrictive and medicine-oriented, and that decision-making must rely on additional forms of evidence. Some researchers argue that EIP provides more flexibility in the nature of the evidence used, and that EIP extends beyond the early definitions of EBP. For this reason, international debate on the utilization of these two concepts is ongoing.

The definition of EIP contains similar components to that of EBP, such as evidence, patient preferences and actions, clinical state and circumstances, and health-care resources. These components are brought together by clinical expertise, through which decisions can be informed.

The term evidence-informed practice has been used, especially in public health and social care. It is defined as: "a complex, multi-disciplinary process that occurs within dynamic and ever-changing communities and encompasses different sectors of society.

Example 4. Evidence-informed Policy Network This is a global WHO initiative that promotes the systematic use of health-research evidence in policymaking and aims to increase Member States' capacity to develop health policy that is informed by research evidence. The network is key in supporting implementation of the European policy framework, Health 2020, and provides a good example of collaboration among countries on utilizing evidence to inform health policies.

The evidence-informed approach continues to evolve as understanding and expertise increase. Some authors promote use of the term EIP to emphasize that the decisionmaking process is person-centred rather than solely focused on scientific research, which, it has been claimed, has taken the humanity out of clinical practice. Both approaches, however, recognize the importance of considering patients/clients' individual needs, unique values, preferences, and circumstances in addition to the scientific evidence that supports and informs clinical decision-making.

Benefits of EBP:

The number of research studies that strive to describe the benefits of making evidence based decision-making standard practice in health systems is vast. EBP is a complex phenomenon, and it is difficult to prove direct causal relationships between the structure of EBP and outcomes in health care. Currently, research mainly focuses on specific interventions and their outcomes. Evidence on the benefits of EBP consequently is mainly indicative. EBP nevertheless has the potential to improve quality of care and produce benefits for patients, nurses and midwives, and the health-care system. It is imperative for countries in the WHO European Region to consider the benefits of EBP and focus on continuous improvement in quality of care.

Benefits for the general population

Implementing EBP creates the conditions for patient-centered care including patient preferences in the decision-making process ultimately has a positive impact on the outcomes of care and health promotion. Successful implementation of EBP enables patients to experience quality health-care services (quality of care is the degree to which health services for individuals and population increase the likelihood of desired health outcomes and are consistent with current professional knowledge) with better outcomes and increased safety (patient safety is defined as the absence of preventable harm to a patient during the process of health care).

Benefits for nurses and midwives Health professionals' strong belief in the value of EBP correlates with increased levels of EBP implementation, job satisfaction and group cohesion. Nurses and midwives who believe in their ability to deliver high-quality care may feel more empowered in their roles and may experience increased cohesion in team structures as they strive towards a common goal of EBP. Continual development of nurses' and midwives' skills in EBP can help them integrate patient preferences into practice and deliver patient-centered care.

Working environments that lack EBP and prevent nurses from reaching their full potential do not support the continued professional growth of nurses, which may result in lower nurse satisfaction and lower compliance with best nursing practices. Nurses and midwives play a crucial role in surveillance and coordination activities that reduce adverse patient outcomes, so are key professionals in improving healthcare quality. Health systems should promote a systematic preventative approach to reducing risks associated with unsafe care and adverse events that ultimately may cause harm to patients. Simply identifying patient safety issues is not sufficient: there is also a need to implement EBP and create a health-care culture that promotes continuous development.

Benefits for health-care systems

The Member States of the WHO European Region, including those with limited healthcare expenditure and which lack effective health-care system structures, can benefit from EBP. The benefits of EBP in countries with insurance-based health-care systems are well known, and health-care providers are being incentivized to implement EBP through mechanisms such as pay for performance.

Health systems can benefit directly from EBP through overall improvement in the quality of care; this means better patient outcomes and increased patient safety. EBP can create economic benefits through reductions in health-care costs.

Health systems that invest in education programmes to improve nurses' and midwives' skills in EBP may benefit from lower turnover rates and greater nurse and midwife satisfaction, resulting in cost savings. This is important for Member States to consider: many countries are currently characterized as having shortages of nurses and midwives, which can ultimately have an adverse impact on the health and well-being of populations.

Improvement in health-care quality enables the development of a healthier, and consequently more productive, population. EBP is not just another highly advanced and extremely expensive western innovation, but an approach that can assist countries experiencing desperate health situations to develop creative and innovative solutions that ultimately benefit patients. EBP interventions can provide policy-makers with reliable evidence and tools on which to base their health-care investment decisions. Organizational leaders who work in under-resourced environments can build capacity for EBP and improve practice through international collaboration, improvement in research networks, and creative and innovative approaches that engage staff to utilize evidence.

Benefits for research and education

Necessary resources for research and development must be allocated to address the research-to-practice gap. As EBP becomes a standard of care, increased production and synthesis of robust evidence in nursing and midwifery will be needed. Nursing and midwifery have their own body of knowledge to guide decision-making in clinical practice. Implementation of EBP is complex and requires much more than simply utilizing research in daily practice. Member States should strive to share knowledge of good practices and support each other in implementing EBP.

EBP has contributed to a major paradigm shift in health-care education and practice. Nurses' and midwives' competence in analysing the best available evidence prior to making recommendations for change in nursing practice has developed over time. The integration of nursing and midwifery expert roles in health-care organizations continues to be of vital importance. These experts, along with researchers, can design and undertake studies that help nurses and midwives make evidence-based decisions on how to prevent health problems or address existing problems. Future health-care professionals need to be sufficiently prepared to work in health-care environments that strive to enable evidence-based decision-making by professionals to be integrated in daily practice. This requires EBP and its related concepts to be incorporated into the education curricula of nursing and midwifery programmes.

common care decisions to improve care processes and patient outcomes.

EBP is one of the programme's six curricular themes, with an EBP module in each year or level of study. Following a progressive pathway, students are initially introduced to scientific enquiry and the role of EBP in nursing. They then learn about types of evidence in EBP in nursing, how to source research articles using key databases, and how to read and understand journal articles. Students develop their literature-searching and scientific-writing skills and are supported in investigating topics with a global or public health focus.

Students acquire a range of research and scholarly skills, which they are encouraged to apply to their clinical learning experiences and theoretical studies as they progress through the programme. They exit the programme as graduate nurses who possess critical reading skills for quantitative and qualitative research evidence to support change in practice, and an appreciation of involving patients in shared decision-making for best possible outcomes.

Example 8. Incorporating EBP into education EBP is incorporated into education at Cardiff University School of Healthcare Sciences, United Kingdom (Wales), in several ways. It is an integral part of undergraduate programmes, and students at master's level have an option of undertaking a systematic review or work-based (implementation) project for their MSc dissertation. The professional doctorate programme also includes a mandatory systematic review module: this is currently being revalidated to incorporate implementation science to encourage students to consider how to put synthesized evidence into practice.

Implementing EBP in nursing and midwifery

New innovations and practices are presented to improve outcomes in nursing and midwifery. Health-care innovation can include the introduction of a new concept, idea, service, process or product that aims to improve treatment, diagnosis, education, outreach, prevention and research, with the long-term goal of improving quality, safety, outcomes, efficiency and costs.

Innovations in health care can be divided into products, processes, and structures. Products typically consist of technology or services, such as clinical procedures. A process refers to a new change to the production or delivery of care. Structures usually affect the internal and external infrastructure of health-care organizations and create new structural models. To be called an innovation, an idea must be replicable and satisfy a specific need. Innovations must have sound scientific justification to be facilitators of EBP. In other words, careful consideration of expected and unexpected outcomes and effectiveness based on current evidence is required when presenting new innovations, such as technology, in nursing and midwifery practice. Implementation should be encouraged for innovations that have proven feasible, appropriate, effective, and meaningful.

Several models have been developed to facilitate the implementation of change in health care. Models and frameworks are used to illustrate EBHC and EBP. Models can be targeted towards specific phases of EBP, focusing on the organization or practitioner. Some (such as Jordan et al.) are generic models that describe the whole process of EBP from research to practice. Others focus on organizational features that support EBP or implementation of evidence throughout the system. The models are not the main point in the development process but are facilitators of change. Models that support organizational change are particularly useful tools for improving and developing EBP.

Currently, an abundance of scientific knowledge is communicated through journals, databases, and so-called grey literature. Cooperation is therefore needed to critically evaluate and synthesize current research into systematic reviews and clinical practice guidelines. International collaborators such as Cochrane and the JBI have developed methodologies for evidence synthesis of different types of research to support the implementation and dissemination of evidence. In addition, multiple national organizations produce systematic reviews, clinical-practice guidelines and methodological guidance for evidence synthesis.

Example 12. JBI collaborating centres in Europe

Example 9. JBI collaborating centres in Europe. The 15 JBI collaborating centres in Europe (2017) synthesize evidence and produce systematic reviews and implementation reports. The Wales Centre for Evidence Based Care, for example, a JBI centre of excellence, focuses on conducting evidence synthesis and teaching healthcare professionals how to undertake comprehensive systematic reviews. The centre is also working with a local health board on a project to implement research findings at local level. centres in Europe

International cooperation, along with national improvements, creates structures that support the development of EBHC and make evidence available for transfer and implementation. There is nevertheless a need to reform management practices in healthcare services at national, regional and local levels towards supporting the development of evidence-based nursing and midwifery.

This requires the creation of specific national, regional and local structures in the following areas to:

- **produce, disseminate, and implement knowledge**
- **develop consistent practices**
- **ensure the continuing development of nurses' and midwives' competence.**

The continuous development of EBP

The development or improvement of a certain health-care practice in an organization requires identification of the current practice, knowledge needs and potential barriers and obstacles to change.

It is imperative that a good understanding of the problem and target group is acquired. The planning of a complex change needs to take into account the specific healthcare context, nature of the innovation and characteristics of the professionals and patients involved. Organizational readiness is the state of preparedness for change, which requires the necessary knowledge, skills, resources, and support. The analysis of organizational readiness can be categorized into organizational culture, infrastructure, and resources. A *(75)*. **Example 12. JBI collaborating centres in Europe**
The awareness stage requires nurse management to increase awareness through enhanced communication, marketing, a monitoring system, and alerts for new information. This results in increased awareness among nurses and midwives. The diffusion of innovation model can be used within the field of nursing to enhance the adoption of innovation relating to EBP. Dissemination of the innovation occurs in the agreement stage of the awareness-to adherence model. Dissemination is the "targeted distribution of information and intervention materials to a specific public health or clinical practice audience".

In this stage, management should present a clear rationale for the innovation, which includes the risks, benefits and associated costs, and staff members' knowledge, attitudes and beliefs about the innovation should be assessed. The adoption and adherence stages involve implementing the change into daily practice. Implementation is the "use of strategies to adopt and integrate evidence-based health interventions and change practice patterns within specific settings". To enhance adoption and adherence, management should provide clear instructions on the desired change, strive to promote consistent practices and inform stakeholders of changes. Leaders should strive to motivate, train and provide incentives to staff members. Management should have a plan for continuous evaluation of outcomes. Adherence routinely occurs for only an estimated one third of evidence in the awareness to-adherence model. It is important to consider the complexity of adoption of EBP when planning an innovation. Successful adoption and sustainability of EBP requires its adoption by individual care providers, leaders and policy-makers. Individual team members cannot support and sustain EBP practices successfully on their own: a collaborative approach is necessary. It is important that management, along with nurses and midwives, identify their roles and responsibilities in the process of EBP development and in sustaining a culture that supports EBP. systematic reviews and implementation reports. The Wales Centre for Evidence Based Care, for

Success factors

It is essential for nurse and midwife managers to commit to the development of consistent nursing and midwifery practice. The use of evidence-based nursing and midwifery guidelines, systematic reviews and recommendations require a new way of thinking, with recognition of the most reliable available evidence that can be applied to clinical practice. Collaboration between health-care organizations and education institutions is a prerequisite to promoting nurses' and midwives' competence in EBP.

Staff competence and their understanding of the basic principles of EBP are important success factors for the implementation of EBP in health care. Improvement opportunities should be offered to staff members so they can take part in developmental work, such as evidence synthesis and implementation projects that facilitate EBP and improve practice and other activities that influence patient outcomes. All actors, however, should have specified roles in the development of EBP to guarantee seamless collaboration.

The essential success factors for implementing and maintaining a successful EBP infrastructure.

1.**generative organization culture,**

2.**shared governance,**

3. **mentors,**

4. **feedback of outcomes,**

5. **visible leadership and support, and**

6. **continuous evaluation of care outcomes.**

7.**Educational programmes**

8.**Tools for dissemination9.Library resources and clinical librarians aching healthcare**

professionals how to undertake comprehensive systematic reviews. The Success factors for EBP include integrating the use of EBP mentors in practice. Mentors play a significant role in implementation through their belief in EBP and ability to engage frontline staff. Shared governance consists of involving and accounting for frontline staff members' perceptions of commitment to, and implementation of, EBP. Staff should be encouraged to participate in EBP projects and decisions that affect the care they provide. Successful EBP infrastructure also requires attention to library resources and clinical librarians, tools for dissemination, multidisciplinary working and educational programmes to ensure successful implementation of EBP.

The ultimate goal of promoting EBP and innovation in health care is to ensure the delivery of equitable, affordable, patient-centred and high-quality health-care services to the entire population. EBHC aims to improve the health and safety of patients while providing care in a cost-effective manner to improve outcomes for patients and health systems. Based on this guide, the following recommendations are offered to support successful development of EBP in nursing and midwifery. .a local health board on a project to implement research findings at local level *(75)*.Th5 JBI collaborating centres in Europe (2017 figure) *(74)* synthesize evidence and produce

systematic reviews and implementation reports. The Wales Centre for Evidence Based Care, for

REFERENCES

1. European strategic directions for strengthening nursing and midwifery towards Health 2020 goals. Copenhagen: WHO Regional Office for Europe; 2015 (http://www.euro.who.int/en/health-topics/Health-systems/nursing-and-midwifery/publications/2015/european-strategic-directions-for-strengthening-nursing-and-midwifery-towards-health-2020-goals, accessed 2 July 2017).

2. Quality of care: a process for making strategic choices in health systems. Geneva: World Health Organization; 2006 (http://apps.who.int/iris/handle/10665/43470, accessed 2 July 2017).

3. Pearson A, Jordan Z, Munn Z. Translational science and evidence-based healthcare: a clarification and reconceptualization of how knowledge is generated and used in healthcare. Nurs Res Pract. 2012;1–6. doi:10.1155/2012/792519.

4. Stevens K. The impact of evidence-based practice in nursing and the next big ideas. Online J Issues Nurs. 2013;18(2):4. doi:10.3912/OJIN.Vol18No02Man04.

5. Jun J, Kovner CT, Stimpfel AW. Barriers and facilitators of nurses' use of clinical practice guidelines: an integrative review. Int J Nurs Stud. 2016;60:54–68. doi:http://dx.doi.org.pc124152.oulu.fi:8080/10.1016/j.ijnurstu.2016.03.006.

6. Scott K, McSherry R. Evidence-based nursing: clarifying the concepts for nurses in practice. J Clin Nurs. 2009;18(8)1085– 95. doi:10.1111/j.1365-2702.2008.02588.x.

7. Spector N. Evidence-based nursing regulation: a challenge for regulators. J Nurs Regul. 2010;1(1):30–6.

8. Jordan Z, Lockwood C, Aromataris E, Munn Z. The JBI model for evidence-based healthcare: a model reconsidered. Adelaide: The Joanna Briggs Institute; 2016 (http://joannabriggs.org/assets/docs/approach/The_JBI_Model_of_Evidence_-_Healthcare-A_Model_Reconsidered.pdf, accessed 2 July 2017).

9. Pearson A, Wiechula R, Court A, Lockwood C. The JBI model of evidence- based healthcare. Int J Evid Based Healthc. 2005;3(8):207–15.

10. Khangura S, Konnyu K, Cushman R, Grimshaw J, Moher D. Evidence summaries: the evolution of a rapid review approach. Syst Rev. 2012;10(1):10. doi:10.1186/2046-4053-1-10.

11. Institute of Medicine. Clinical practice guidelines we can trust. Washington (DC): National Academies Press; 2011.

12. Enabling breastfeeding for mothers and babies. In: Cochrane Library Special Collection [website]. London: The Cochrane Collaboration; 2017 (http://www.cochranelibrary.com/app/content/special-collections/ article/?doi=10.1002/14651858.10100214651858, accessed 2 July 2017).

13. WHO, Facilitating evidence-based practice in Nursing & Midwifery. http://www.euro.who.int

8. GENETICS AND GENETIC COUNCELLING

Genetics is the branch of science concerned with genes, heredity, and variation in living organisms. It seeks to understand the process of trait inheritance from parents to offspring, including the molecular structure and function of genes, gene behaviour in the context of a cell or organism (e.g., dominance and epigenetics), gene distribution, and variation and change in populations.

A history of genetics and genomics

Genetics is the study of heredity, which means the study of genes and factors related to all aspects of genes. The scientific history of genetics began with the works of Gregor Mendel (**the father of Genetics)** in the mid-19th century. Prior to Mendel, genetics was primarily theoretical whilst, after Mendel, the science of genetics was broadened to include experimental genetics. Developments in all fields of genetics and genetic technology in the first half of the 20th century provided a basis for the later developments. In the second half of the 20th century, the molecular background of genetics has become more understandable. Rapid technological advancements, followed by the completion of Human Genome Project, have contributed a great deal to the knowledge of genetic factors and their impact on human life and diseases. Currently, more than 1800 disease genes have been identified.

Importance of medical genetics

- 50% of first trimester abortion are due to chromosomal abnormalities
- Congenital malformation: 2-3% of newborns.
- 2% infants are born with single gene disorder
- More than half of childhood blindness, deafness and mental retardation are due to genetic disorders.

SUBDIVISIONS OF GENETICS

The four major subdivisions of Genetics

---

1. **Classical Genetics**
2. **Molecular Genetics**
3. **Population Genetics**
4. **Quantitative Genetics**

---

1. **Classical genetics:** Study of transmitting traits from generation to generation and physical traits as a stand-in or the genes that control appearance, or phenotype.

2. **Molecular genetics:** The chemistry of genes which investigate the structures and functions of genes at the molecular level. Investigate the physical and chemical structures of the double helix, DNA and how the genetic code works at the levels of DNA and RNA

3. **Population genetics:** The use of Mathematics and equations to describe what goes on genetically is population genetics. Its use of Mendelian genetics and examine the inheritance patterns of many different individuals who have something like geographic location in common.

4. **Quantitative genetics:** Measuring the strength of heredity and examines traits that vary in subtle ways and relates those traits to the underlying genetics of organisms. It works on a complex statistical approach to estimate how much variation in a particular trait is due to the environment.

Genetic information

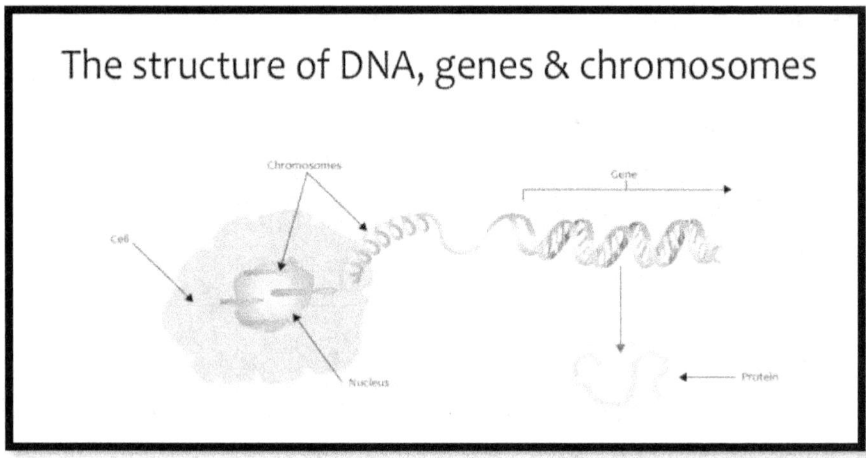

Figure 35: Structure of DNA, gene & Chromosomes

Chromosomes

They are thread-like structures in which nucleic acids and protein found in the nucleus of most living cells, carrying genetic information in the form of genes. DNA is tightly packaged within the nucleus. DNA is coiled around proteins called histones. As they are storage units of genes.

- Chromatin: DNA, RNA & proteins that make up chromosome.
- Chromatids: one of the two identical parts of the chromosome.
- Centromere: the point where two chromatids attach
- Pairs: 46 chromosomes. 22 pairs Autosomes and 1 pair Sex chromosomes.

Nucleotide

Group of molecules that when linked together, form the building blocks of DNA and RNA; composed of phosphate group, the bases: adenosine, cytosine, guanine and thymine and a pentose sugar. In case of RNA, thymine base is replaced by uracil.

Codon

Series of three adjacent bases in one polynucleotide chain of a DNA or RNA molecule which codes for a specific amino acid.

Gene

The functional and physical unit of heredity passed from parent to offspring. Genes reside on chromosomes. If a gene is like a chapter in a book, the chromosome is the book itself. Proteins and RNA influence how an organism looks, how well its body metabolizes food and fights infection, and even how it behaves.

Genome

The entire DNA contains in an organism or a cell which is the collection of genetic information.

DNA (deoxyribonucleic acid) – It is a nucleic acid that contains the genetic instructions specifying the biological development of all cellular forms of life. It is a double-stranded molecule made up of four building blocks called nucleotide bases (different chemicals that are abbreviated A(Adenine) T(Thymine) C(Cytosine) and G(Guanine) that are arranged in a certain order throughout a genome

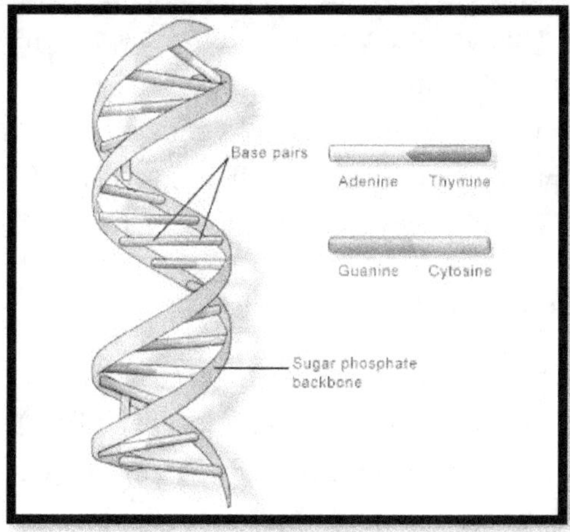

Figure 36: Structure of DNA

Genetic concept

Genetic Concepts: Chromosome - double stranded DNA molecule packaged by histone & scaffold proteins

Chromosome numbers constant for an organism

- n - haploid number
- 2n – diploid number
- Each individual inherits 23 chromosomes from father and 23 from mother.
- Humans: 2n= 46 chromosomes
- Humans 23 paternal, 23 maternal
- Each maternal & paternal pair represent homologous chromosomes - called homologs

Haploid or Homologous Chromosomes:

- Share centromere position
- Share overall size
- Contain identical gene sets at matching positions (loci) gene for color gene for shape

Diploid:

- Diploid organisms contain 2 alleles of each locus (gene)
- Alleles can be identical – homozygous
- Alleles can be different – heterozygous
- If only one allele is present – hemizygous – Case in males for genes on X and Y chromosomes

Medal's law of inheritance

Humans have long bred plants and animals to favour certain traits (e.g., dogs that retrieve things, trees that produce a lot of fruit). Thus, we know that these traits are influenced by genes. Such traits (called complex traits) vary continuously, like a bell curve, from less to more.

Complex Traits

The specific degree of a complex trait is very difficult to predict from one generation to the next (e.g., the exact height of offspring). This is because the precise combination of genes contributing to the trait cannot be predicted either (or, perhaps, even known). When geneticists look for evidence of genetic influence on a disease, such as heart disease or mental illness, they look for families that have many affected over several generations.

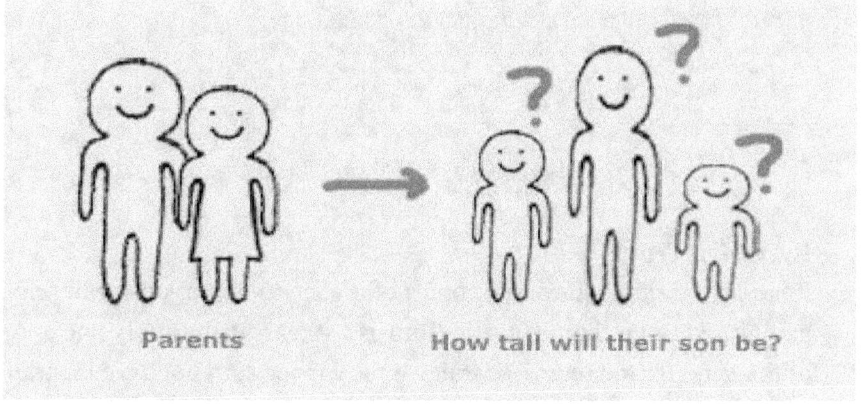

Figure 37: Complex Traits

Dominant Traits

Unlike common complex traits, certain rare traits do show clear patterns of inheritance. In these traits, single genes strongly influence a trait in an 'either/or' manner. Dominant traits require only one copy of a gene to express the trait (e.g., ability to roll your tongue, Huntington disease).

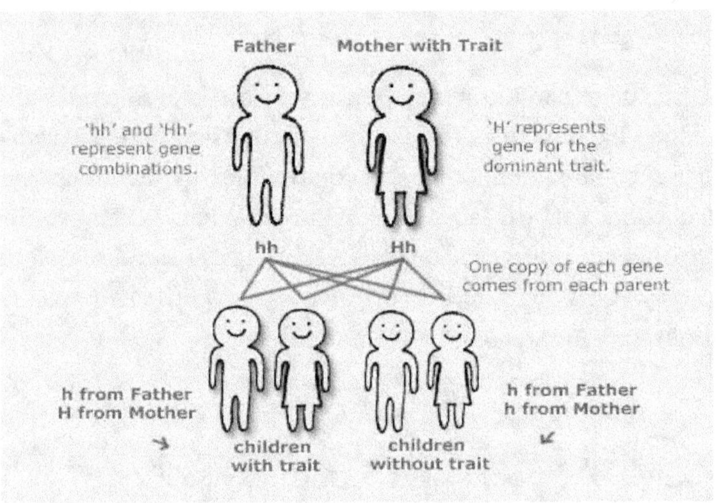

Figure 38: Dominant Traits

Recessive Traits

Recessive traits require two copies of a gene to express the trait (e.g., having a straight thumb, cystic fibrosis). A 'carrier' has only one copy of the gene for the recessive trait, so the carrier does not have the trait.

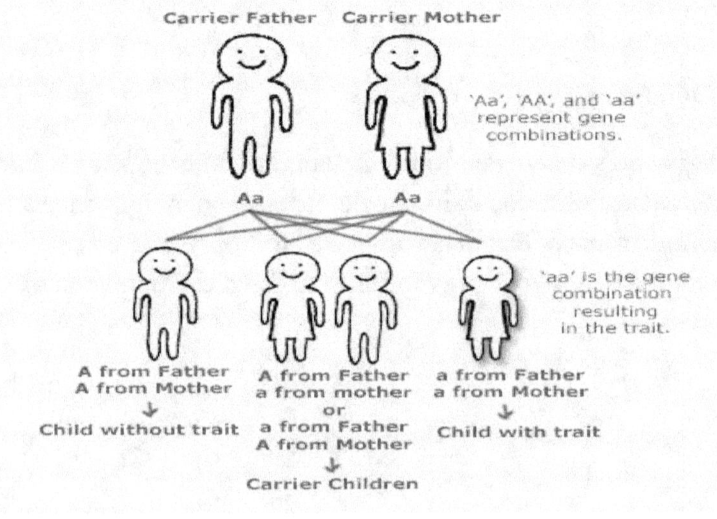

Figure 39: Recessive Traits

Patterns of inheritance

Medical Genetics studying rare disorders, 4 general patterns of inheritance are observed:

1. Autosomal recessive

The disease appears in male and female children of unaffected parents. e.g., Sickle cell anaemia, Phenylketonuria

2. Autosomal dominant

Affected males and females appear in each generation of the pedigree. Affected mothers and fathers transmit the phenotype to both sons and daughters, e.g., Neurofibromatosis, Adult polycystic kidney disease.

3. X-linked recessive

Many more males than females show the disorder. All the daughters of an affected male are "carriers". None of the sons of an affected male show the disorder or are carriers; e.g., Haemophilia , Colour blindness

4. X-linked dominant

Affected males pass the disorder to all daughters but to none of their sons. Affected heterozygous females married to unaffected males pass the condition to half their sons and daughters, e.g. Vitamin D resistant rickets.

5. Codominant inheritance

Two different versions (alleles) of a gene can be expressed, and each version makes a slightly different protein. Both alleles influence the genetic trait or determine the characteristics of the genetic condition. e.g., ABO locus (The ABO locus encodes three alleles, that is, 3 variants of the same gene. One allele is derived from each parent)

6. Mitochondrial inheritance

This type of inheritance applies to genes in mitochondrial DNA Mitochondrial disorders can appear in every generation of a family and can affect both males and females, but fathers do not pass mitochondrial traits to their children. e.g., Leber's hereditary optic neuropathy (LHON).

MUTATION

Definition:

Permanent changes in the DNA. Those that affect germ cells are transmitted to the progeny. Mutations in the somatic cells are not transferred to the progeny but are important in the causation of cancer and some congenital diseases.

Causes Of Mutation

- **Chemicals**
- **Nitrous acid**
- **Alkylating agents**
- **5-bromouracil**
- **Antiviral drug iododeoxy uridine**
- **Benzopyrene in tobacco smoke**
- **X – rays & ultraviolet light**
- **Certain viruses such as bacterial virus**

Types Of Mutations -

point mutation, change within a gene in which one base pair in the DNA sequence is altered. Point mutations are frequently the result of mistakes made during DNA replication, although modification of DNA, such as through exposure to X-rays or to ultraviolet radiation, also can induce point mutations. It is categorized as

Silent mutation: It is non-expressive. In silent mutation, a new codon codes for the same amino acid as the wild-type one. Mis-sense mutation: A codon originated from a nucleotide change that will code for different amino acids. It can lead to alteration or loss of function in protein.

Nonsense mutation: A stop codon is added to the premature protein. It stops protein synthesis because a stop codon ends synthesis of protein and results in a premature protein or truncated protein.

Frameshift mutation: Base pair alteration causes abnormal reading frame which ultimately results in an abnormal protein formation. A specific reading frame has a start codon and a stop codon. In between both codons, a definite coding sequence is present. In a frameshift mutation, alteration in DNA leads to shifting of this reading frame from one place to another in a genome.

Trinucleotide Repeat Mutations: set of genetic disorder caused by trinucleotide repeat in certain genes exceeding normal, stable threshold e.g., Fragile X Syndrome.

GENETIC DISORDERS

A genetic disease is any disease caused by an abnormality in the genetic makeup of an individual. The genetic abnormality can range from minuscule to major -- from a discrete mutation in a single base in the DNA of a single gene to a gross chromosomal abnormality involving the addition or subtraction of an entire chromosome or set of chromosomes. Some people inherit genetic disorders from the parents, while acquired changes or mutations in a preexisting gene or group of genes cause other genetic diseases. Genetic mutations can occur either randomly or due to some environmental exposure.

Types Of Genetic Disorders (Inherited)

There are a number of different types of genetic disorders (inherited) and include:

1. **Single gene inheritance**
2. **Multifactorial inheritance**
3. **Chromosome abnormalities**
4. **Mitochondrial inheritance**

1. **Single gene inheritance:**

Single gene inheritance is also called Mendelian or monogenetic inheritance. Changes or mutations that occur in the DNA sequence of a single gene cause this type of inheritance. There are thousands of known single-gene disorders. These disorders are known as monogenetic disorders (disorders of a single gene).

Single-gene disorders have different patterns of genetic inheritance, including

- Autosomal dominant inheritance, in which only one copy of a defective gene (from either parent)
- Autosomal recessive inheritance, in which two copies of a defective gene (one from each parent)
- X-linked inheritance, in which the defective gene is present on the female, or X-chromosome. X-linked inheritance may be dominant or recessive.

Some examples of single-gene disorders include

- **Cystic fibrosis,**
- **Alpha- and beta-thalassemia**
- **Sickle cell anemia (sickle cell disease),**
- **Marfan syndrome,**
- **Fragile X syndrome,**
- **Huntington's disease,**
- **Hemochromatosis.**

---

2. **Multifactorial inheritance:** Multifactorial inheritance is also called complex or polygenic inheritance. Multifactorial inheritance disorders are caused by a combination of environmental factors and mutations in multiple genes. For example, different genes that influence breast

cancer susceptibility have been found on chromosomes 6, 11, 13, 14, 15, 17, and 22. Some common chronic diseases are multifactorial disorders.

Examples of multifactorial inheritance include

- **Heart Disease,**
- **High Blood Pressure,**
- **Alzheimer's Disease,**
- **Arthritis,**
- **Diabetes,**
- **Cancer,**
- **Obesity.**

Multifactorial inheritance also is associated with heritable traits such as fingerprint patterns, height, eye color, and skin color.

3. **Chromosome abnormalities:** Chromosomes, distinct structures made up of DNA and protein, are located in the nucleus of each cell. Because chromosomes are the carriers of the genetic material, abnormalities in chromosome number or structure can result in disease. Chromosomal abnormalities typically occur due to a problem with cell division. For example, Down syndrome (sometimes referred to as "Down's syndrome") or trisomy 21 is a common genetic disorder that occurs when a person has three copies of chromosome 21. There are many other chromosomal abnormalities including:
   - Turner syndrome (45, X0)

     It, a condition that affects only females, results when one of the X chromosomes (sex chromosomes) is missing or partially missing. Turner syndrome can cause a variety of medical and developmental problems, including short height, failure of the ovaries to develop and heart defects.

- Klinefelter syndrome (47, XXY)

  It is **a genetic condition affecting males**, and it often isn't diagnosed until adulthood. Klinefelter syndrome may adversely affect testicular growth, resulting in smaller than normal testicles, which can lead to lower production of testosterone.

- Cri du chat syndrome, or the "cry of the cat" syndrome (46, XX or XY, 5p-).

  It is a syndrome, also known as 5p- (5p minus) syndrome, is **a chromosomal condition that results when a piece of chromosome 5 is missing**. Infants with this condition often have a high-pitched cry that sounds like that of a cat.

4. **Mitochondrial inheritance:** This type of genetic disorder is caused by mutations in the non-nuclear DNA of mitochondria. Mitochondria are small round or rod-like organelles that are involved in cellular respiration and found in the cytoplasm of plant and animal cells. Each mitochondrion may contain 5 to 10 circular pieces of DNA. Since egg cells, but not sperm cells, keep their mitochondria during fertilization, mitochondrial DNA is always inherited from the female parent.

Examples of mitochondrial disease include

- Leber's hereditary optic atrophy (LHON), an eye disease;
- Myoclonic epilepsy with ragged red fibers (MERRF); and
- Mitochondrial encephalopathy, lactic acidosis, and stroke-like episodes (MELAS), a rare form of dementia.

GENETIC COUNSELLING

Genetic counselling is a service that provides information and advice about genetic condition. These are condition caused by changes known as mutation in certain genes and are usually passed down through a family.

Genetic counselling is the process through which knowledge about the genetic aspects of illnesses is shared by trained professionals with those who are at an increased risk or either having a heritable disorder or of passing it on to their unborn offspring. A genetic counsellor   provides information on the inheritance of illnesses and their recurrence risks; addresses the concerns of patients, their families, and their health care providers; and supports patients and their families dealing with these illnesses. The Heredity Clinic was the first genetic counselling service centre established in 1940 at the University of Michigan, USA. Since then, the many such centers have been opened around the world.

Genetic counselling may be described as the process through which individuals affected by, or at risk for a problem which may be genetic or hereditary, are informed of the consequences of the disorder, of the probability of suffering from or of transmitting it to their offspring, and of the potential means of treating or of avoiding the occurrence of the malformation or disease in question. Genetic counselling in common disorders is often given by the family doctor, the paediatrician or the obstetrician. However, with the recognition that thousands of problems have a major hereditary component, counselling is increasingly done in specialized centres which also provide the laboratory diagnostic tools.

History and evolution of genetic counseling

"Sheldon Clark Reed" coined the term genetic counselling in 1947 and published the book **"Counselling in Medical Genetics"** in 1955. Most of the early genetic counselling clinics were run by non-medical scientists or by those who were not experienced clinicians. With the growth in knowledge of genetic disorders and the appearance of medical genetics as a distinct specialty in the 1960s, genetic counselling progressively became medicalized, representing one of the key components of clinical genetics. It was not, though, until later that the importance of a firm psychological basis was recognized and became an essential part of genetic counselling, the writings of Seymour Kessler making a particular contribution to this. The first master's degree genetic counselling program in the United States was founded in 1969 at Sarah Lawrence College in Bronxville, New York. In 1979, the National Society of Genetic Counsellors (NSGC) was founded

Definition

Genetic counselling is a communication process, which aims to help individuals, couples and families understand and adapt to the medical, psychological, familial, and reproductive implications of the genetic contribution to specific health conditions. A communication process that deals with human problems associated with the occurrence or the risk of occurrence of genetic disorders in individuals or families. Genetic counselling is communicative process which deals with human problems associated with occurrence and or recurrence of a genetic disorder in a family

Aims of genetic counseling

The genetic counselling aims to provide the family with complete and accurate information about genetic disorders.

1. Promoting informed decisions by involved family members
2. Clarifying the family's options available treatment and prognosis
3. Explaining alternatives to reduce the risk of genetic disorders
4. Decreasing the incidence of genetic disorders
5. Reducing the impact of the disorders

Purpose of genetic counseling

- **Explaining alternatives to reduce the risk of genetic disorders.**
- **Reducing the impact of genetic disorders.**
- **Assisting families in choosing the options most appropriate for them.**
- **To comprehend the medical facts, including diagnostic and available management. Discussing the options available for dealing with the disorder.**
- **Provide concrete, accurate information about inherited disorders.**

- **Reassure people who are concerned that their child may inherit a particular disorder**
- **Allow people who are affected by inherited disease to make informed choice about future.**
- **Educate people about inherited disorder and the process of inheritance.**
- **Offer support by skilled health care professionals to people who are affected by genetic.**
- **To comprehend the medical facts, including diagnostic, probable course of the disorder**
- **To appreciate the way hereditary contributes.**
- **To understand the option for dealing with the risk occurrence.**
- **Possible adjustment to the disorder in an affected family member.**

Indications of genetic counselling

1. **Advanced parental age:**
   - Maternal age $\geq$35 yrs
   - Paternal age $\geq$50 yrs
2. **Previous child with or family H/O:**
   - Hereditary disease in a patient or family
   - Congenital anomaly
   - Dysmorphism
   - Intellectual disability
   - Developmental delay
   - Isolated birth defect
   - Metabolic disorder
   - Chromosomal abnormality
   - Myopathy/ Neuropathy
   - Ambiguous genitalia

3. **Adult-onset genetic disorder (pre symptomatic testing)**
   - Cancer - Inherited a tendency to develop cancer
4. Consanguinity - Couples are blood relatives.
5. Teratogen exposure
6. Repeated pregnancy loss or infertility
7. Pregnancy screening abnormality

- **Maternal serum α-foeto protein**
- **Maternal triple or quad test**
- **Fetal ultrasonography**
- **Fetal karyotype**

---

8. **Heterozygote screening based on ethnic risk**
   - Sickle cell anemia
   - Tay- Sachs, Canavan, Gaucher disease
   - Thalassemia
9. Follow up to abnormal neonatal genetic testing
10. Other Indication:

- **Birth defects**
- **Mental retardation**
- **Miscarriages**
- **Malformations**
- **Tendency to develop a neurologic condition**
- **Birth defects and genetic condition.**
- **Child with defects / genetic condition.**
- **Child with developmental delay**
- **Mental retardation and other problems with growth and developments.**

Types of genetic counselling

They are of 2 types:

Prospective genetic counselling:

This allows for the true prevention of disease. This approach requires

- Identifying heterozygous individuals for any defect by screening
- Explaining to them the risk of their having affected children if they marry another heterozygote for the same gene.
- If heterozygous marriage can be prevented or reduced, the prospects of giving birth to affected children will diminish. EX: Sickle cell anemia Thalassemia

Retrospective genetic counselling:

- Most genetic counselling at present is retrospective, i.e, the hereditary disorder has already occurred within the family.
- The methods which could be suggested under retrospective genetic counselling are: Contraception and Pregnancy termination.

Types of genetic screening

A search in apparently normal population for individual with abnormal genes which increase their risk or their offspring of being affected by a disease.

1. **Carrier identification**

   It is possible to identify the healthy carriers of a number of genetic disorders, especially the inborn errors of metabolism

2. **Prenatal diagnosis**

   Prenatal diagnosis forms an integral step in genetic counselling. In fact, for couples at risk of a disorder, it is desirable to consider, plan and discuss prenatal diagnosis even before pregnancy. Discussion and planning beforehand will eliminate hurried procedures and emotional trauma as well.

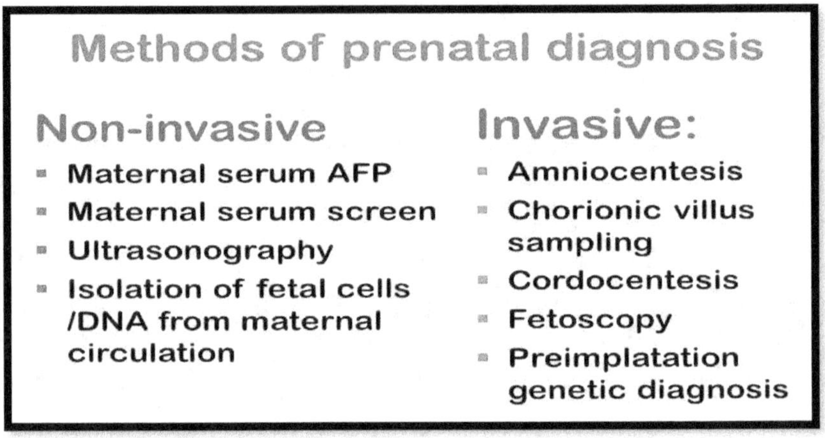

Figure 40: Approaches to prenatal diagnosis

3. Newborn screening

Newborn screening is the practice of testing all babies in their first days of life for certain disorders and conditions that can hinder their normal development. This testing is required in every state and is typically performed before the baby leaves the hospital.

Forensic screening (paternity test)

Paternity tests consist of determining the genetic maps that belong to the two people who undergo the analysis. By comparing the genetic map of the suspected father with that of the child, it is possible to determine their biological kinship.

Steps of genetic counselling

- Diagnosis-based on accurate family History
- Examination and Investigation
- Risk assessment
- Communication
- Discussion of Options
- Long-term contact and support

Diagnosis-based on accurate family history

This is primary beginning phase of counselling in which following tasks are accomplished

- Initial interview with counselee & family for preparation of counselee for counseling.
- Carryout primary assessment of counselee, physical examination etc.
- Considering potential diagnosis based on collected information.

Examination & Investigation

- Most crucial step in any genetic consultation; involves History taking, Examination and Investigation
- In some cases, the goal of genetic evaluation is to make a diagnosis of genetic condition/ syndrome.
- In other cases, the diagnosis already is known, and the genetic counselor probably will confirm the established diagnosis to proceed for next phases of the counseling.
- There are two investigations are said to done as follows:

---

1. **Confirmatory /Supplementing Tests**
   a. **Chromosomal analysis**
   b. **Biochemical tests**
   c. **Molecular DNA testing**
   d. **X Rays, biopsy**
   e. **Immunological test**
   f. **Prenatal diagnosis**
   g. **Linkage analysis**
2. **Establishment of an Accurate Diagnosis**

Risk Assessment

This phase includes followings tasks.

- Literature search and review of information.
- Consultation with other experts.
- Compiling of information and determination of recurrence risk.

Communication

- Communication of results and risk to the counselee and to the family if appropriate.
- Discussion of natural history of disorders.
- Current treatment options and anticipatory guidance.
- Assess the counselee's understanding about facts and relevant hereditary pattern, diagnostic and management options for disorder.

Discussion of Option

- Consultants should be provided with all of the information necessary for them to make their own informed decisions.
- It should include details of all the options available
- If relevant, the availability of prenatal diagnosis should be discussed, together with details of the techniques, limitations and risks associated with the various methods employed
- Various reproductive options –donor sperm, donor ova or PGD

Long Term Contact and Support:

- It should present information clearly in sympathetic and appropriate manner
- It be receptive to the fears and aspirations, expressed or unexpressed
- The setting should be agreeable, private and quiet, with ample time for discussion and questions
- Technical terms should be avoided or, if used, fully explained
- Questions should be answered openly and honestly
- Written summary for follow up
- Should contact the consultant at later date
- Should refer to appropriate patient support groups

Pre-requisites of genetic counselling

- Detailed family history.
- Accurate diagnosis.
- Understanding medical aspect of disorder (etiology, history, treatment, prognosis, burden).
- Understanding the inheritance pattern (recurrence risk)
- Understanding the psycho-social impact of the information.
- Training / experience in counselling techniques.
- Understanding the concepts of health / disease / healthcare in the appropriate cultures.

Role of nurses/midwives in genetic counselling

- **Receive the client and family and make them comfortable in assessment room for genetic counseling.**
- **Obtain prenatal, family, and other health histories from individual and family.**
- **Conduct primary physical information and collect other relevant information.**
- **Provide psychological support to individual and family throughout the counseling.**
- **Provide information about hereditary pattern.**
- **Collect other relevant information from individual and family e.g. – any prior test report and documents others.**
- **Encourage the individual and other family members to ask questions as much as they can understand about all aspects of disorders.**
- **Establish a plan of care with the family and coordination care with the family and other healthcare professionals.**
- **Maintain privacy and confidentiality of all the information.**
- **Provide referral guidance.**
- **Follow up care**

Role of genetic counselor

- Educate individuals, families, and communities about inheritance, testing, management, prevention, resources, and research in genetic counseling.
- Explain family history and the chance that a condition will occur or recur.
- Counsel an individual or family to promote informed choices and adaptation to the risk or condition.

Importance of Genetic counselling in Maternal and Child Health

In India, birth defects prevalence varies from 61 to 69.9/ live births. Major birth defects include congenital heart defects, neural tube defects, Down syndrome, haemoglobinopathies and glucose -6- phosphate dehydrogenase deficiency, cause 20% of infant mortality and are responsible for childhood hospitalizations. It has been estimated that 70% of birth defects are preventable by prenatal genetic counselling. Advances in genetic science have increased the number of health interventions. Genetics is therefore expanding into the domain of national screening programmes, disease prediction and pharmacogenetics. This expansion means that health professionals especially midwives, need skill and knowledge in genetics in order to take new roles. Educational provision on genetic for midwives is insufficient. Genetic education for midwives is an important strategy which facilitates pregnant women to discuss their concerns with midwives to understand better about genetic testing and disorders that can be detected and refer women to specialist services thereby reduce the infant mortality and enhance mother and child welfare.

REFERENCE

1. https://www.medicinenet.com/breast_cancer_pictures_slideshow/article.html
2. https://www.ashg.org/education/everyone_1.shtml
3. https://www.news-medical.net/life-sciences/What-is-enetics.aspx
4. https://www.nature.com/subjects/genetics
5. Autosomal Dominant Disorder, https://www.genome.gov
6. Huntington's Disease, https://www.ninds.nih.gov
7. Structure of Chromosomes, https://www.n.gov

www.ingramcontent.com/pod-product-compliance
Lightning Source LLC
LaVergne TN
LVHW041321200726
843509LV00009B/567